Case-Based Studies in Cardiac Electrophysiology

Editors

LUIGI DI BIASE
EMILY P. ZEITLER

CARDIAC ELECTROPHYSIOLOGY CLINICS

www.cardiacep.theclinics.com

Consulting Editors
LUIGI DI BIASE
EMILY P. ZEITLER

June 2024 • Volume 16 • Number 2

ELSEVIER

1600 John F. Kennedy Boulevard • Suite 1800 • Philadelphia, Pennsylvania, 19103-2899

http://www.theclinics.com

CARDIAC ELECTROPHYSIOLOGY CLINICS Volume 16, Number 2
June 2024 ISSN 1877-9182, ISBN-13: 978-0-443-29348-1

Editor: Joanna Gascoine
Developmental Editor: Shivank Joshi

Cardiac Electrophysiology Clinics (ISSN 1877-9182) is published quarterly by Elsevier Inc., 360 Park Avenue South, New York, NY 10010-1710. Months of issue are March, June, September, and December. Subscription prices are $262.00 per year for US individuals, $286.00 per year for Canadian individuals, $348.00 per year for international individuals, and $100.00 per year for US, Canadian and international students/residents. For institutional access pricing please contact Customer Service via the contact information below. To receive student/resident rate, orders must be accompanied by name of affilliated institution, date of term, and the signature of program/residency coordinator on institution letterhead. Orders will be billed at individual rate until proof of status is received. Foreign air speed delivery is included in all Clinics subscription prices. All prices are subject to change without notice. **POSTMASTER:** Send address changes to Cardiac Electrophysiology Clinics, Elsevier Health Sciences Division, Subscription Customer Service, 3251 Riverport Lane, Maryland Heights, MO 63043. **Customer Service: 1-800-654-2452 (US and Canada). From outside of the US and Canada, call 314-477-8871. Fax: 314-447-8029. E-mail: JournalsCustomerService-usa@elsevier.com (for print support); JournalsOnlineSupport-usa@elsevier.com (for online support).**

Reprints. For copies of 100 or more of articles in this publication, please contact the Commercial Reprints Department, Elsevier Inc., 360 Park Avenue South, New York, NY 10010-1710. Tel.: 212-633-3874; Fax: 212-633-3820; E-mail: reprints@elsevier.com.

Cardiac Electrophysiology Clinics is covered in *MEDLINE/PubMed (Index Medicus)*.

Contributors

CONSULTING EDITORS

LUIGI DI BIASE, MD, PhD, FACC, FESC, FHRS
Section Head of Electrophysiology, Director of Arrhythmia Services, Professor of Medicine (Cardiology), Montefiore-Einstein Center for Heart and Vascular Care, Montefiore Medical Center, Albert Einstein College of Medicine, Bronx, New York, USA

EMILY P. ZEITLER, MD, MHS, FHRS
Cardiac Electrophysiology, Assistant Professor of Medicine, The Geisel School of Medicine at Dartmouth, Hanover, New Hampshire, USA; Dartmouth Health, Assistant Professor of Health Care Policy, The Dartmouth Institute, Dartmouth Hitchcock Medical Center, Lebanon, New Hampshire, USA

EDITORS

LUIGI DI BIASE, MD, PhD, FACC, FESC, FHRS
Section Head of Electrophysiology, Director of Arrhythmia Services, Professor of Medicine (Cardiology), Montefiore-Einstein Center for Heart and Vascular Care, Montefiore Medical Center, Albert Einstein College of Medicine, Bronx, New York, USA

EMILY P. ZEITLER, MD, MHS, FHRS
Cardiac Electrophysiology, Assistant Professor of Medicine, The Geisel School of Medicine at Dartmouth, Hanover, New Hampshire, USA; Dartmouth Health, Assistant Professor of Health Care Policy, The Dartmouth Institute, Dartmouth Hitchcock Medical Center, Lebanon, New Hampshire, USA

AUTHORS

JOSE AGUILERA, MD
Cardiac Electrophysiology Fellow, Section of Cardiac Pacing and Electrophysiology, Heart and Vascular Institute, Cleveland Clinic, Cleveland, Ohio, USA

MUTAZ ALKALBANI, MBBS
Fellow, Inova Schar Heart and Vascular, Falls Church, Virginia, USA

AYSHA ARSHAD, MD, FACC, FHRS, FAHA
Clinical Cardiac Electrophysiologist, Inova Schar Heart and Vascular, Falls Church, Virginia, USA; Carient Heart and Vascular, Manassas, Virginia, USA

TOMMASO BARBATI, MS
Texas Cardiac Arrhythmia Institute, St. David's Medical Center, Austin, Texas, USA

ULRIKA BIRGERSDOTTER-GREEN, MD
Division of Cardiology, Section of Electrophysiology, University of California San Diego, La Jolla, California, USA

JUAN CABRERA, MD
Section of Electrophysiology, Fundación Cardioinfantil, Bogotá, Colombia

STEPHANIE F. CHANDLER, MD
Assistant Professor, Division of Cardiology, Ann & Robert H. Lurie Children's Hospital of Chicago, Northwestern University Feinberg School of Medicine, Chicago, Illinois, USA

LUIGI DI BIASE, MD, PhD, FACC, FESC, FHRS
Section Head of Electrophysiology, Director of Arrhythmia Services, Professor of Medicine (Cardiology), Montefiore-Einstein Center for Heart and Vascular Care, Montefiore Medical

Center, Albert Einstein College of Medicine, Bronx, New York, USA

MOHAMMAD A. EBRAHIM, MD
Department of Pediatrics, Chest Diseases Hospital, Kuwait University, Kuwait City, Kuwait

SUSAN P. ETHERIDGE, MD
Professor, Department of Pediatrics, Division of Cardiology, University of Utah and Primary Children's Hospital, Salt Lake City, Utah, USA

KIROLLOS GABRAH, DO
Arrhythmia Research Group, Jonesboro, Arkansas, USA

CAROLA GIANNI, MD
Texas Cardiac Arrhythmia Institute, St. David's Medical Center, Austin, Texas, USA

RADY HO, MD
Cardiologist, Lehigh Valley Heart and Vascular Institute, Allentown, Pennsylvania, USA

SAMI H. IBRAHIM, MD
Cardiology Fellow, University of Virginia, Charlottesville, Virginia, USA

EFEHI IGBINOMWANHIA, MD, MPH
Fellow, Heart and Vascular Institute, MetroHealth Medical Center, Case Western Reserve University, Cleveland, Ohio, USA

IGNACIO INGLESSIS-AZUAJE, MD
Director Adult Congenital Heart Disease Interventions, Corrigan Minehan Heart Center, Massachusetts General Hospital, Boston, Massachusetts, USA

SANIA JIWANI, MD
Fellow, Department of Cardiovascular Medicine, University of Kansas Medical Center, Kansas City, Kansas, USA

SUNIL KAPUR, MD
Staff Cardiac Electrophysiologist, Brigham and Women's Hospital, Boston, Massachusetts, USA

SAIMA KARIM, DO
Cardiologist, Heart and Vascular Institute, MetroHealth Medical Center, Case Western Reserve University, Cleveland, Ohio, USA

SUJOY KHASNAVIS, MD
Jacobi North Central Bronx Medical Center, Albert Einstein College of Medicine, Bronx, New York, USA

ANDREW KRUMERMAN, MD, FHRS
Professor of Medicine, Montefiore-Einstein Center for Heart and Vascular Care, Montefiore Medical Center, Bronx, New York, USA

VINCENZO MIRCO LA FAZIA, MD
Texas Cardiac Arrhythmia Institute, St. David's Medical Center, Austin, Texas, USA

ANNE-SOPHIE LACHARITE-ROBERGE, MD
Fellow, Division of Cardiology, Section of Electrophysiology, University of California San Diego, La Jolla, California, USA

VICTORIA LUU, BA
Carient Heart and Vascular, Manassas, Virginia, USA

ARUN UMESH MAHTANI, MD, MS
Resident, Arrhythmia Research Group, Department of Internal Medicine, Jonesboro, Arkansas, USA

PAMELA K. MASON, MD, FHRS, FACC
Professor of Medicine, Director, Electrophysiology Laboratory, University of Virginia, Charlottesville, Virginia, USA

MELANIE MAYTIN, MD, MSc
Physician, Cardiovascular Medicine, Brigham and Women's Hospital, Boston, Massachusetts, USA

THEOFANIE MELA, MD
Cardiac Electrophysiologist, Corrigan Minehan Heart Center, Massachusetts General Hospital, Boston, Massachusetts, USA

CHRISTINA Y. MIYAKE, MD, MS
Assistant Professor, Department of Pediatrics, Division of Cardiology, Texas Children's Hospital, Baylor College of Medicine, Houston, Texas, USA

SANGHAMITRA MOHANTY, MD
Director, Translational Research, Texas Cardiac Arrhythmia Institute, St. David's Medical Center, Austin, Texas, USA

DEVI G. NAIR, MD, FACC, FHRS
Director, Arrhythmia Research Group,
Department of Electrophysiology, St. Bernards
Medical Center, Jonesboro, Arkansas, USA

ANDREA NATALE, MD
Executive Medical Director, Texas Cardiac
Arrhythmia Institute, St. David's Medical
Center, Austin, Texas, USA

MARY C. NIU, MD
Department of Pediatrics, Division of
Cardiology, University of Utah, Primary
Children's Hospital, Salt Lake City, Utah, USA

VIDISH PANDYA, MD
Resident Physician, Department of Medicine,
Montefiore Medical Center, Bronx, New York,
USA

KAVISHA PATEL, MD
Fellow, Division of Cardiology, Section of
Electrophysiology, University of California San
Diego, La Jolla, California, USA

NILAY PATEL, MD
Corrigan Minehan Heart Center,
Massachusetts General Hospital, Boston,
Massachusetts, USA

TAM DAN PHAM, MD
Assistant Professor, Department of Pediatrics,
Texas Children's Hospital, Houston, Texas,
USA

RHEA PIMENTEL, MD
Associate professor, Department of
Cardiovascular Medicine, University of Kansas
Medical Center, Kansas City, Kansas, USA

TRAVIS L. POLLEMA, DO
Division of Cardiovascular and Thoracic
Surgery, University of California San Diego, La
Jolla, California, USA

LUIS CARLOS SAENZ, MD
Director, International Arrhythmia Center,
Section of Electrophysiology, Fundación
Cardioinfantil, Bogotá, Colombia

RAHUL SAKHUJA, MD
Interventional Cardiologist, Corrigan Minehan
Heart Center, Massachusetts General
Hospital, Boston, Massachusetts, USA

PASQUALE SANTANGELI, MD, PhD
Associate Section Head and VT Program
Director, Section of Cardiac Pacing and
Electrophysiology, Heart and Vascular
Institute, Cleveland Clinic, Cleveland, Ohio,
USA

SAMER SAOUMA, MD
Clinical Cardiac Electrophysiology Fellow,
Montefiore Medical Center, Albert Einstein
College of Medicine, Bronx, New York, USA

THOMAS M. TADROS, MD
Cardiovascular Medicine, Brigham and
Women's Hospital, Boston, Massachusetts,
USA

MARTIN TRISTANI-FIROUZI, MD
Professor, Department of Pediatrics,
Division of Cardiology, University of Utah,
Primary Children's Hospital, Salt Lake City,
Utah, USA

GREGORY WEBSTER, MD, MPH
Section Chief, Electrophysiology. Assistant
Professor of Pediatrics (Cardiology), Division of
Cardiology, Ann & Robert H. Lurie Children's
Hospital of Chicago, Northwestern University
Feinberg School of Medicine, Chicago, Illinois,
USA

YANG YANG, MD
Fellow, Division of Cardiology, Section of
Electrophysiology, University of California San
Diego, La Jolla, California, USA

XIAODONG ZHANG, MD, PhD
Assistant Professor, Department of Medicine
(Cardiology), Montefiore Medical Center, Albert
Einstein College of Medicine, Bronx, New York,
USA

FENGWEI ZOU, MD
Fellow, Montefiore-Einstein Center for Heart
and Vascular Care, Montefiore Medical Center,
Bronx, New York, USA

Contents

Transvenous laser lead extraction poses a risk of major complications (0.19%–1.8%), notably injury to the superior vena cava (SVC) in 0.19% to 0.96% of cases. Various factors contribute to SVC injury, which can be categorized as patient-related (such as female gender, low body mass index, diabetes, renal problems, anemia, and reduced ejection fraction), device-related (including the number, dwell time, and type of leads), or procedural-related (such as reason for extraction, venous obstructions, and bilateral lead placements).

The population of patients with advanced heart failure continues to increase steadily as does the need for mechanical circulatory support. Combination therapy with left ventricular assist devices (LVADs) and cardiovascular implantable electronic devices (CIEDs) is unavoidable. CIED complications in patients with LVADs are common and often necessitate device system revision and transvenous lead extraction. Despite this, management recommendations are limited, and guidelines are lacking.

 Video content accompanies this article at http://www.cardiacep.theclinics.com.

Persistent left superior vena cava (PLSVC) is an anatomic variant that is relatively uncommon in the general population. Lead extraction through PLSVC is extremely rare. Due to unusual anatomy, the procedure carries challenges that require special considerations and careful planning. The authors report a case of lead extraction through a PLSVC with occluded right superior vena cava and highlight the challenges and outcomes of the procedure.

This case report discusses a 42-year-old male with dextro-transposition of the great arteries (D-TGA) status post Mustard repair and sick sinus syndrome status post dual-chamber pacemaker implant, who developed symptomatic superior vena cava (SVC) baffle stenosis. He was treated with a combined pacemaker extraction and subsequent SVC baffle stenting. The case highlights the complexities of treating SVC baffle stenosis in the presence of cardiac implantable devices and demonstrates the efficacy of this combined approach. Furthermore, the authors delve into the intricacies of D-TGA, its surgical history, and the long-term complications associated with atrial switch procedures.

 Video content accompanies this article at http://www.cardiacep.theclinics.com.

We present a complex case of cardiac implantable electronic device infection and extraction in the setting of bacteremia, large lead vegetation, and patent foramen ovale. Following a comprehensive preprocedural workup including transesophageal echocardiogram and computed tomography lead extraction protocol, in addition to the involvement of multiple subspecialties, an open chest approach to extraction was deemed a safer option for eradication of the patient's infection. Despite percutaneous techniques having evolved as the preferred extraction method during the last few decades, this case demonstrates the importance of a thorough evaluation at an experienced center to determine the need for open chest extraction.

Leadless pacemaker systems (LPs) were developed as an alternative to traditional transvenous permanent pacemakers (TV-PPM) due to increasing rates of device and procedural related complications, leading to a high-cost burden to our healthcare system. LPs were initially indicated for single-chamber ventricular pacing; however, recent developments have allowed for dual-chamber pacing too. These systems have demonstrated highly successful implant rates with stable pacing performance. This article describes the retrieval techniques of the Micra LPs and ways to mitigate challenges encountered during the retrieval process.

Cardiac implantable electronic device leads can contribute to tricuspid regurgitation and also complicate surgical and transcatheter interventions to manage tricuspid regurgitation. Here we present a case of a patient with sinus node dysfunction and complete heart block who underwent extraction of a right ventricular pacing lead before tricuspid valve surgery. We review the data regarding the contribution of leads to tricuspid regurgitation and the benefits of lead extraction, risks of jailing leads during tricuspid interventions, and pacing considerations around tricuspid valve procedures.

A 69-year-old woman with a history of heart failure with reduced ejection fraction presented for device interrogation of her cardiac implantable electronic device (CIED), revealing lead and pulse generator displacement. Surprisingly, she exhibited a narrow QRS on the ECG despite an underlying right bundle branch block, suggesting unintentional conduction system pacing (CSP). Traditional cardiac resynchronization therapy has been widely used for patients with heart failure, but alternatives like CSP are emerging as viable options. Given the global rise in CIED utilization, regular follow-up, device troubleshooting, and embracing remote monitoring are essential to manage and optimize patient outcomes.

A 34-year-old woman presented with palpitations and paroxysmal atrial fibrillation (AF). Workup revealed anterior mitral valve prolapse with severe mitral regurgitation. She was referred for surgical repair and underwent a mitral valve replacement, tricuspid valve repair, and bi-atrial cryoMAZE procedure with left atrial appendage ligation. Her postoperative course was complicated by inferior wall myocardial infarction. She subsequently presented with palpitations and underwent electrophysiology study and ablation. This case illustrates pitfalls associated with the surgical MAZE procedure and highlights the challenges in postoperative atrial arrhythmias diagnosis and management.

 Video content accompanies this article at http://www.cardiacep.theclinics.com.

The left atrial appendage (LAA) is now recognized as a significant contributor to arrhythmia and thromboembolism in patients with a history of atrial fibrillation. Thoracoscopic exclusion of the LAA is made possible with the AtriClip device. In this report, we describe the case of a 65-year-old man with history of multiple left atrial ablation procedures and LAA clipping. He developed a microreentrant atrial tachycardia originating from the anterior base of the LAA stump, underwent complete isolation of the LAA, and had subsequent resolution of arrhythmogenic activity from the residual LAA stump.

A 70-year-old man with recurrent atrial fibrillation (AF) underwent transcatheter radiofrequency ablation after an earlier unsuccessful attempt. Although typical AF triggers were ablated, the patient's condition persisted, leading to the identification of the interatrial septum (IAS) as the probable source of the tachycardia trigger. Given the depth and thickness of the IAS, traditional radiofrequency ablation proved ineffective. However, using the alternative method of bipolar radiofrequency catheter ablation (B-RFCA), the atrial tachycardia was successfully terminated. B-RFCA demonstrates potential for effectively terminating tachycardias originating from deep intramural locations, suggesting its potential as a pivotal technique for complex cases with septal atrial tachycardia.

 Video content accompanies this article at http://www.cardiacep.theclinics.com.

The epicardial outflow tract can be a site of origin of idiopathic ventricular arrhythmias. These arrhythmias are most commonly perivalvular and can be targeted from within the coronary venous system or from other adjacent structures, such as the right ventricular and left ventricular outflow tracts or the coronary cusp region. The authors report a case of an epicardial idiopathic outflow tract premature ventricular contraction originating from the midseptal epicardial left ventricle. In this case, direct epicardial access was crucial to identify early local activation and achieve successful catheter ablation.

The case series reviews differential diagnosis of a genetic arrhythmia syndrome when evaluating a patient with prolonged QTc. Making the correct diagnosis requires: detailed patient history, family history, and careful review of the electrocardiogram (ECG). Signs and symptoms and ECG characteristics can often help clinicians make the diagnosis before genetic testing results return. These skills can help clinicians make an accurate and timely diagnosis and prevent life-threatening events.

Bidirectional ventricular tachycardia is a unique arrhythmia that can herald lethal arrhythmia syndromes. Using cases based on real patient stories, this article examines 3 different presentations to help clinicians learn the differential diagnosis associated with this condition. Each associated genetic disorder will be briefly discussed, and valuable tips for distinguishing them from each other will be provided.

The following case series presents three different pediatric patients with *SCN5A*-related disease. In addition, family members are presented to demonstrate the variable penetrance that is commonly seen. Identifying features of this disease is important, because even in the very young, SCN5A disorders can cause lethal arrhythmias and sudden death.

CARDIAC ELECTROPHYSIOLOGY CLINICS

SERIES OF RELATED INTEREST

Cardiology Clinics
https://www.cardiology.theclinics.com/
Interventional Cardiology Clinics
https://www.interventional.theclinics.com/
Heart Failure Clinics
https://www.heartfailure.theclinics.com/

THE CLINICS ARE AVAILABLE ONLINE!
Access your subscription at:
www.theclinics.com

Foreword
Challenge Accepted

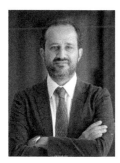 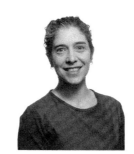

Luigi Di Biase, MD, PhD, FACC, FESC, FHRS   Emily P. Zeitler, MD, MHS, FHRS
Consulting Editors

The field of scientific inquiry is led by brave minds who think the unthinkable and do the undoable. Thanks to those pioneers, the field of cardiac electrophysiology has witnessed dramatic evolution since its inception. More than 60 years ago, the first transvenous pacemaker was implanted in humans. Today, electrophysiology is a field that encompasses advanced pacing strategies, such as cardiac resynchronization, conduction system pacing and leadless pacing, the ability to map and ablate complex atrial and ventricular tachyarrhythmias using a variety of energy sources, and many more. As versatile as our toolbox is, we continue to encounter complex clinical scenarios of cardiac arrhythmias that challenge the preexisting understanding of anatomy, pathophysiology, and treatment. We are pleased to introduce this issue of the *Cardiac Electrophysiology Clinics* that focuses on complex ablation of atrial and ventricular arrhythmias, device management, lead extraction, and genetics of cardiac electrophysiology through a series of cases. Case reports introduce us to the newest challenges in the field

and reflect a "first try" at a problem. They also tickle the reader's brains on how they would solve the clinical conundrum if they were taking care of the patient described. Case reports are where new technologies are first reported. So, sit back and enjoy this packed issue of interesting and intriguing cases.

Luigi Di Biase, MD, PhD, FACC, FESC, FHRS
Albert Einstein College of Medicine
at Montefiore Health System
New York, NY 10467, USA

Emily P. Zeitler, MD, MHS, FHRS
Dartmouth Health Lebanon, New Hampshire
The Dartmouth Institute
Lebanon, New Hampshire, USA

The Geisel School of Medicine at Dartmouth
Hanover, New Hampshire, USA

E-mail addresses:
dlbbla@gmail.com (L. Di Biase)
Emily.p.zeitler@hitchcock.org (E.P. Zeitler)

Preface

Case-Based Studies in Cardiac Electrophysiology

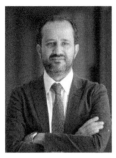 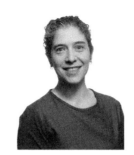

Luigi Di Biase, MD, PhD, FACC, FESC, FHRS   Emily P. Zeitler, MD, MHS, FHRS
Editors

One of the most fascinating aspects of practicing clinical medicine is that no matter how experienced a clinician is, there are always patients who present with unusual problems or ordinary problems with unusual symptoms. These cases are often not well studied and inspire us to go back to the basics, revisit physiology and anatomy, and think outside the box. Reporting complex cases not only demonstrates the limitations of current understanding of disease but also proposes new areas for discussion and discovery. In parallel we are exposed to new technologies on a regular basis. Notable examples in recent years include pulsed-field ablation as a novel energy source that has the potential to change how we perform catheter ablation, conduction system pacing as step towards approximating native conduction, and many more. As we embrace these new advances, trial and error through experience is a necessary process that allows operators to fully understand how to apply these technologies safely and effectively.

In this issue of *Cardiac Electrophysiology Clinics*, we present a series of cases that underscores challenges of current practice in cardiac electrophysiology, innovative approaches and techniques to procedures, and outlooks for generating hypotheses to continue pushing the field forward. In the section on complex ablation, contributors offer cases of both atrial and ventricular tachyarrhythmias. These cases not only emphasize the importance of careful mapping in patients with complex history but also explore how a new generation of tools is used to conquer difficult anatomy. In the section on device and lead management, the contributing authors delve into complex extraction as life expectancy increases and modern devices are more versatile and complicated. And last but not least, a series of cases highlights how genetics play an important role in the practice of electrophysiology. As we learn from these complex cases, we improve together as a field. Just as Winston Churchill once said: out of intense complexities, intense simplicities emerge.

Card Electrophysiol Clin 16 (2024) xv–xvi
https://doi.org/10.1016/j.ccep.2023.12.004
1877-9182/24/© 2023 Published by Elsevier Inc.

cardiacEP.theclinics.com

DISCLOSURE

Include a disclosure statement with any commercial or financial conflicts of interest and any funding sources for all guest editors.

Luigi Di Biase, MD, PhD, FACC, FESC, FHRS
Albert Einstein College of Medicine at
Montefiore Health System
New York, NY 10467, USA

Emily P. Zeitler, MD, MHS, FHRS
Dartmouth Health Lebanon
New Hampshire
The Dartmouth Institute
Lebanon, New Hampshire, USA

The Geisel School of Medicine at
Dartmouth
Hanover, New Hampshire, USA

E-mail addresses:
dibbia@gmail.com (L. Di Biase)
emily.p.zeitler@hitchcock.org (E.P. Zeitler)

Case Series and Review of Literature for Superior Vena Cava Injury During Laser Lead Extraction

Efehi Igbinomwanhia, MD, MPH[a],*, Sania Jiwani, MD[b], Saima Karim, DO[a], Rhea Pimentel, MD[b]

KEYWORDS

- Multidisciplinary approach to laser lead extraction • Incidence of superior vena cava injury
- Risk factors for superior vena cava injury • Superior vena cava bridge balloon utilization

KEY POINTS

- Superior vena cava injury during transvenous lead extraction is rare, but causes significant morbidity and mortality.
- Patient-related, device-related, and procedure-related risk factors may contribute to complications due to transvenous lead extractions, including superior vena cava injury.
- Perioperative preparation with a multidisciplinary team approach is essential in the timely management of superior vena cava injury during transvenous lead extraction.

INTRODUCTION

Transvenous laser lead extraction has a major complication rate reported in the range of 0.19% to 1.8% and minor complication rate reported in the range of 0.6% to 6.2%[1] (**Tables 1** and **2**). Lead extraction requires preparation and coordination between multiple teams to avoid poor outcomes and expeditiously treat complications. The most feared complication is a superior vena cava (SVC) or SVC-right atria junction (SVC-RA) injury. The rate of vascular laceration during lead extraction ranges from 0.19% to 0.96%.[1] Procedural planning includes assessment of high-risk patient and device characteristics with preoperative imaging and blood work. Cardiothoracic surgery (CTS) consultation can be instrumental in the workup of the patient. During the procedure, certain measures can be employed preemptively to manage complications in the event of an SVC or SVC-RA injury. CTS backup availability and expedient surgical management of vascular complications can decrease mortality. The authors review two cases involving SVC tears and various methods deployed in preparation for lead extraction.

CASES

Case 1

A 57-year-old woman with a history of tobacco abuse, and syncope due to complete heart block with dual-chamber Medtronic pacemaker was seen in clinic for persistently elevated right ventricular (RV) threshold and battery status indicating elective replacement indicator (ERI). Patient had Medtronic right atrial (RA) lead (model 5068, length 52 cm) and the RV lead (model 5068, length 58 cm) implanted 21 years ago with latest generator being 8 year old (Medtronic, model ADDRL1). After discussion of risks, benefits, and options, she opted to move forward with a transvenous lead extraction (TLE) and generator change. Her transthoracic

[a] Heart and Vascular Institute, MetroHealth Medical Center/Case Western Reserve University, 2500 Metrohealth Drive, Cleveland, OH 44109, USA; [b] Department of Cardiovascular Medicine, University of Kansas Medical Center, 3901 Rainbow Boulevard, Mailstop 4023, Kansas City, KS 66160, USA
* Corresponding author. Heart and Vascular Institute, MetroHealth Medical Center, 2500 Metrohealth Drive, Cleveland, OH 44109.
E-mail address: eigbinomwanhia@metrohealth.org

Card Electrophysiol Clin 16 (2024) 117–124
https://doi.org/10.1016/j.ccep.2023.10.011
1877-9182/24/Published by Elsevier Inc.

Table 1
Risk factors for transvenous lead extraction dependent on patient characteristics, device characteristic, and procedure-specific risk factors

Patient-related factors	
Female sex	• Higher risk of major complications[2,6–9]
BMI <25 kg/m^2	• Higher risk of major adverse events as well as in-hospital[3] and 30-d all-cause mortality[10]
Diabetes mellitus	• Higher in-hospital all-cause mortality[3]
Renal dysfunction	• Creatinine $\geq$2.0 mg/dL: Higher in-hospital all-cause mortality[3] • End stage renal disease: Higher mortality at 1 month and 6 month[11]
Left ventricular dysfunction (ejection fraction <15%)	• Higher rate of major complications[10]
Anemia	• Hemoglobin <11.5 g/dL: Higher odds of major complications • Higher 30-d all-cause mortality[7,12]
Procedural and device factors	
Number of leads extracted	• Higher risk of major complications with $\geq$3 leads extracted[6,13,14]
Implant duration	• 8%–22% higher odds of major complications per 1 year of implant duration[6,15] • Mean lead dwell time of >10 year: Independent predictor for vascular avulsion/tear[15]
Infection as indication for extraction	• Higher rate of complications and 30-d all-cause mortality[6]
Occlusion or critical stenosis of the superior venous access	• Independent predictor for vascular avulsion or tear[16]
Targeted leads on both right and left sides	• Increased risk of complications with laser extraction[9,17]
Dual-coil ICD leads	• More difficult to remove than single-coil ICD leads[18] • Higher 30-d all-cause mortality[10]
Lead diameter, coil shape, proximal coil surface area	• Higher rate of complications with extraction of ICD leads[6]
ePTFE-coated ICD leads	• Shorter procedure times and less need for advanced tools[19,20]

echocardiogram (TTE) showed normal left ventricular (LV) and RV size and function. Non-contrast computerized tomography (CT) obtained showed leads adherent to SVC/RA area, RV lead being at apex, moderate coronary calcification, thoracic aortic calcification, and centrilobular emphysema. CTS and preoperative anesthesia teams were consulted. All anticoagulants were held 5 days before the planned TLE.

After the patient underwent sterile draping and prepping in the hybrid operating room (OR), bilateral femoral venous access was obtained. A Bridge balloon was deployed for appropriate position and then retracted into the inferior vena cava after marking optimal deployment position over the Amplatz wire through a 12-Fr sheath. Other femoral access consisted of a 7-French sheath, through which a temporary backup pacing catheter was placed as patient was atrial-dependent. The femoral sheaths were also connected to a line provided to anesthesia in the event of blood transfusion. Further, an arterial line was placed.

Subsequently, patient underwent laser lead extraction using a #2 lead locking stylet and a 14-French 80 Hz energy Spectranetics laser that was unsuccessful due to significant vascular calcification. Therefore, a mechanical extraction tool was used. Although TLE was performed around the SVC-RA junction, the patient was noted to be hypotensive and had transient pulseless electrical arrest for 2 minutes requiring chest compression. Patient was immediately stabilized after resuscitation. Transesophageal echocardiogram (TEE) showed a moderate loculated effusion by the RV. Blood transfusion was initiated, and laboratory workup was urgently sent. CTS was called as the Bridge balloon was deployed. Via the subclavian vascular access now available, new RV lead (Medtronic 5076, length 58 cm) was placed while awaiting surgical backup.

Table 2
Periprocedural management and preparation for transvenous lead extraction

Periprocedural Management	Description
Risk assessment	Review patient's medical history and lead characteristics Use risk stratification tools
Multidisciplinary team	Involvement of electrophysiologists, cardiac surgeons, anesthesiologists, and support staff preoperatively A cardiac surgeon with the ability to provide emergent thoracotomy in <5 minute should be available[42]
Imaging modality	Chest x-ray, cardiac computed tomography, venography for additional risk assessment can be used[21–27] Transesophageal echocardiography (TEE) or intracardiac echocardiography (ICE) for continuous procedural monitoring[34,35]
Anticoagulation management	Individualize anticoagulation use, taking in account thromboembolic risk[31]
Anesthesia and sedation	General anesthesia with controlled ventilation for most cases given TEE utility in most cases
Vascular access	Plan for large-bore vascular sheaths and femoral access Plan for arterial line for continuous hemodynamic measurement
Endovascular balloon	Balloons for SVC occlusion can be considered[43] May be reasonable to preposition in high-risk cases[44]

CTS arrived within 3 minutes and emergent midline incision sternotomy was performed. Pericardium was opened and good hemostasis was obtained. Proximal control was obtained at the SVC-RA junction along with distal SVC control, while the bridge balloon was still deployed. Clips were deployed over a small branch of the azygous, whereas repair sutures were placed on the posterior aspect of the SVC and the RA junction. There was now reasonable resuscitation of the patient and good control of bleeding. Two temporary ventricular wires were placed and secured as the patient was dependent on pacing. The permanent pacer was set to dual chamber pacing mode with a rate of 60 to 120 beats per minute, and the backup epicardial pacer was set to 40 beats per minute ventricular pacing. The Sternum was packed, and patient was transported back to the ICU in critical, but hemodynamically stable condition.

Case 2

A 66-year-old woman (body mass index [BMI] 24.5 kg/m^2) with a history of supraventricular tachycardia, hypertension, hyperlipidemia, seizure disorder, tobacco abuse, and sinus node dysfunction with placement of Abbott dual-chamber pacemaker 8 years prior presented to the office with atrial lead malfunction and generator at ERI. She was referred for RA removal and reimplantation

with generator change. Device interrogation demonstrated 81% RA pacing and 2.5% RV pacing with intermittent oversensing of RA lead with stable impedance and elevated RV lead thresholds. A decision was made to extract and reimplant both leads after risks and potential complications were discussed with the patient in detail.

Device consisted of Abbott Medical isodiametric 7-French RV (model 1948, length 52 cm, passive fixation) and RA (model 1944, length 46 cm, passive fixation) leads. The outer insulation was composed of polyurethane and silicone. Preoperative TTE showed normal LV function and chest x-ray suggested axillary vein access. CT scan revealed both leads hugged the lateral wall of SVC/RA junction with RV lead terminating in apical septum and RA lead in the RA appendage. The patient underwent CTS and anesthesia consult before procedure. Appropriate blood work was also obtained.

The procedure was performed under general anesthesia in a hybrid OR. Intraoperative baseline TEE before the procedure showed normal LV function and trace pericardial effusion. The patient was prepped and draped, and right femoral arterial and bilateral femoral venous accesses were obtained. An Amplatzer exchange length wire was advanced through the 12-Fr right femoral vein for potential Bridge balloon deployment. A temporary transvenous pacer was also placed. The generator and the leads were dissected out in pocket before disconnection.

Gentle traction on the leads indicated vascular adhesions. A #2 locking stylet was placed to the tip of the RV lead. Using 80-Hz energy, a Spectranetics 14-Fr laser sheath was advanced from the access site to the midportion of the SVC. 40-Hz pulsation was then applied around the SVC/RA junction with gentle traction which released the RV lead from myocardium without any complications, changes in blood pressure, or pericardial effusion.

Next, a #2 locking stylet was inserted in RA lead but could not be advanced beyond the SVC/RA junction due to suspected lead fracture. With a 14-Fr laser, 40-Hz pulsations were used to advance the laser sheath through the SVC/RA junction. The patient remained hemodynamically stable without new pericardial effusion on TEE. Having arrived at the juncture where the locking stylet ended, moderate manual traction on the lead with forward pressure using the laser sheath alone was applied. At this point, there was a rapid drop in the patient's systolic blood pressure from 120 to 50 mm Hg. Cardiopulmonary resuscitation was initiated immediately. Repeat TEE imaging revealed no new pericardial effusion.

CTS was in the control room and activated. Massive transfusion protocol was initiated. While cardiopulmonary resuscitation was continued, the bridge balloon was deployed. CT surgery team performed emergent sternotomy with a large amount of clot noted in pericardium. The patient was placed on a cardiac bypass pump and required cardiac massage for ventricular fibrillation during the transition. An SVC laceration was identified, and primary repair performed. The RA lead was abandoned and clipped at the pocket level. A temporary epicardial wire was placed. The vascular access was oversewn, and chest pocket closed.

Postoperatively, the patient was monitored in the ICU setting. She was gradually weaned off hemodynamic support and extubated. Epicardial pacing lead was removed.

DISCUSSION

Leads from cardiac implantable electronic devices are exposed to continual stress, leading to a finite lifespan. As patient longevity improves with existing devices, a concomitant increase in device complications, including lead malfunction and infection, exists. The long-term risks of simply abandoning leads must be balanced against the risk of complex TLE. TLE is often considered a high-risk procedure, but large observational studies have not borne this out. The most feared risk of extraction is SVC injury often leading to rapid hemodynamic compromise and death. A study of 91,890 TLR procedures identified using the Nationwide Inpatient Sample from 2006 to 2012 showed a 2.0% overall rate of vascular injury with a significant increase in trend over the study period.[2] The LExICon study had a 0.41% rate of vascular tear (including axillary artery tear) requiring thoracotomy, pericardiocentesis, chest tube, or surgical repair.[3] Most SVC tears during TLE occur in the isolated body of the SVC.[4] The recently published retrospective multicenter CLEAR study reported risk factors associated with perforation which include no history of cardiac surgery, female sex, preserved LV ejection fraction, lead age greater than 8 years, ≥2 leads extracted, and diabetes.[5]

The authors discuss the various risk factors for major complications associated with lead extraction, subdividing them into patient characteristics, device characteristics, and procedural characteristics.

PATIENT CHARACTERISTICS

Female sex is associated with a higher risk of procedural complications from TLE in general (especially for high voltage leads) with 1.19 to 2.74 higher odds of complications in multiple studies.[3,6–9] The patient's BMI less than 25 kg/m^2 portends a higher risk of procedure-related major adverse events, in-hospital,[3] and 30-day all-cause mortality.[10] Patients with diabetes mellitus as well as with creatinine ≥2.0 mg/dL have been shown to have a higher rate of in-hospital mortality.[3] End-stage renal disease with dialysis dependency is associated with higher mortality at 1 month (Hazard ratio [HR] 5.60 [2.67–11.53]) and 6 months (HR 2.81 [1.74–4.42]).[11] Also, an ejection fraction of ≤15% correlates with a significantly higher risk of major complication.[10] The presence of anemia with hemoglobin concentration less than 11.5 g/dL is associated with a greater than two times odds of major complications[7,12] and every 1 g/dL lower hemoglobin concentration leads to an increase in major complications by 22.4% to 27.4%.[9] The presence of anemia is also associated with a higher 30-day all-cause mortality odds ratio (OR) 3.3; 95% CI: 2.0–5.0).[10]

PREOPERATIVE DEVICE RISK FACTORS

Device characteristics play a key role in determining procedural risk. The number of leads extracted[6,13] and longer lead implant duration[6,14] are widely recognized risk factors for major complications. The risk of complications is twofold when three or more leads are extracted. The odds of complications increase by 8% to 22% per 1 year of implant duration.[6,15] Leads greater than 10 year old were shown to pose the highest risk with 13 times odds of complications when compared with leads less than 5 year old.[15] A mean lead dwell time of greater than 10 years is an independent risk predictor for vascular avulsion/tear (OR 3.19; 95% CI 1.21–8.40).[16]

The indication for extraction should also be considered. Extraction for infection is associated with a higher rate of complications during TLE (OR 2.27, 95% CI 1.70–3.04).[6] Moreover, in-hospital[3] and 30-day all-cause mortality (OR 2.7; 95% CI: 1.4–5.0)[10] are increased when TLE performed for device infection. It is unclear whether this is due to the overall comorbid disease in a patient with infection. In the ELECTRa registry, the presence of occlusion or critical stenosis of the superior venous access was an independent predictor for vascular avulsion or tear (OR 5.74; 95% CI 1.71–19.22).[16] The presence of targeted leads on both right and left sides of chest increases the risk of acute complications with laser extraction as well (OR 9.4; 95% CI: 1.6–54.3).[17]

Risk factors specific to extraction of high-voltage cardiac leads include smaller lead diameter, flat versus round coil shape, and higher proximal coil surface area.[6] Implantable cardioverter defibrillator (ICD) leads with an SVC coil are 2.6 times more difficult to remove than single-coil ICD leads and associated with a significantly higher rate of complications[18] and a higher 30-day all-cause mortality (OR 2.7; 95% CI: 1.6–4.5).[10] Expanded polytetrafluoroethylene (ePTFE)-coated ICD leads are resistant to fibrosis and often result in shorter procedure times and less need for advanced tools[19,20]

The SAFeTY score was developed to predict the risk of procedural complications and need for surgical backup for TLE. It includes the patient and device characteristics with sum of lead dwell times (S), anemia (A), female sex (Fe), treatment/previous procedures (T), and young patients less than 30 years (Y). A score of ≥10 is considered high risk and is associated with a 2.5% probability of major complications. This increases to greater than 11.82% in very high-risk patients identified by a score of ≥16.[7]

PREOPERATIVE PREPARATION

Preoperative preparation is a critical component of lead extraction procedures. A thorough evaluation of the patient's medical history, comorbidities, device specifics, and current medication is necessary for risk stratification and identifying any potential contraindications that may affect the procedure. Preoperative imaging also plays a crucial role in preoperative preparation and surgical response.

All patients should undergo a chest x-ray, which provides information regarding lead positioning/course, integrity, type of fixation, and lead design. Dual-coil design and passive fixation leads have shown to be associated with more fibrous adhesions.[21] Gated cardiac CT has emerged as a valuable imaging modality to analyze venous stenosis/occlusion, lead positioning/course, lead perforation, lead fracture, and adhesions.[22] The presence of severe lead adhesions (leads with no surrounding contrast or blood) was associated with a more complex procedure, including laser sheath size upgrade, longer fluoroscopic time, femoral snare use, and need for laser and/or mechanical sheath.[22] Patients with higher lead-to-lead binding had more challenging extractions as measured by extraction time and laser pulses.[23] In the recently published MILES study, cardiac CT with higher fibrosis score predicted need for powered sheath during extraction.[24]

Venography can also be used to assess extent of lead adhesions. Long adherent segments have been associated with longer fluoroscopy time and need for power tools.[25] In addition, lead-related venous stenosis or occlusion on venography is associated with higher risk of lead fracture during extraction, longer procedure time, need for different venous approach, lead-to-lead adhesion, increased extraction complexity. and the use of metallic sheaths and femoral tools.[26]

In suspected CIED infection, TEE can aid with the detection of intracardiac thrombi/vegetations and concomitant tricuspid valvular disease. Open surgical extraction to mitigate thromboembolic risk if large vegetations (>3.0 cm) present should be considered.[27]

Renal function, coagulation, and hemoglobin levels should be obtained preoperatively. Patients suspected of having CIED infection should be on the appropriate antibiotics. Anticoagulation management decisions should be made in conjunction with CTS. A previous observational study reported up to 1.3 increased risk of death and a threefold increased risk of major complications in patients with elevated international normalised ratio (INR).[10] However, others have demonstrated safety of uninterrupted warfarin with therapeutic INR and with direct acting oral anticoagulants (DOAC) during extraction.[28–30] Anticoagulation protocol during TLE should consider predictors of thrombotic events such as the presence of mechanical valve prostheses, atrial fibrillation. The current consensus guidelines recommend that anticoagulant management be reassessed on a case-by-case basis.[31]

PROCEDURAL PHASE

Patients should undergo sterile preparation in case an emergent sternotomy is required, ensuring a sterile field encompasses the entire front of the chest and femoral regions. Two to four units of packed red blood cells should be immediately available, especially in cases with higher complication risk.[31]

An arterial line should be placed to enable invasive blood pressure monitoring and femoral central access obtained to ensure prompt resuscitative measures in case of SVC tear.[32,33] Continuous TEE-guided TLE use can increase rates of complete procedural success and reduce risk of severe complications, ultimately preventing periprocedural deaths.[34] TEE also aids in monitoring hemodynamics, adjusting vasoactive medications and promptly identifies complications leading to a timelier intervention. Intracardiac echocardiography (ICE) has emerged as another valuable tool in TLE for demonstrating fibrotic areas, lead adhesions, and presence of any remaining lead fragments or remnants. However, the use of ICE during extraction requires a second operator and its presence in the RA may limit space for necessary tools.[35] Shockwave intravascular lithotripsy is a novel technique that was recently explored as an adjunct to pretreat vessels with dense calcification via shock wave therapy. It was shown to reduce procedural time by 25 minutes.[36]

There are no established guidelines regarding the ideal setting (such as an electrophysiology suite or hybrid OR) for TLE, nor are there specific recommendations regarding the level of surgical backup needed. Common practices include selection of low-risk patients for electrophysiology suite, whereas moderate to high-risk candidates may undergo TLE in the hybrid suite or OR.[15,37–40] The shoulder-to-shoulder approach (co-operator with a cardiac surgeon) has been shown to improve procedural success but with no mortality benefit.[41,42] Regardless of the setting, TLE should be done in a location that will allow for emergent sternotomy or thoracotomy within 5 to 10 minutes of a complication.[42]

In the event of an SVC tear or injury, it is crucial to stabilize the patient in preparation for emergency surgical repair. The use of endovascular occlusion balloon can serve as a bridging technique. Extraction complicated by SVC tear with successful deployment of occlusion balloon was associated with an 87% reduction of in-hospital mortality.[43] Another emerging practice in the use of endovascular balloon is the preemptive deployment of the balloon to enable rapid advancement and inflation of the balloon in the event of an SVC tear, thus reducing deployment time by 90 seconds and saving appropriately 700 cc of blood loss.[44] It should be noted that the balloon utility is limited to extra pericardial injury of a limited size because if there is injury greater than 80 mm (length of the balloon), there will be incomplete occlusion.[43] Cardiopulmonary bypass can also be used to transiently stabilize a patient during an SVC tear especially when femoral access has been secured.

Overall, the preoperative and intraoperative measures used increase the risk of success and survival while improving response times in the rare cases that surgical backup is required during a TLE. These preparations are best served when protocolized by individuals and institutions to increase the success of lead extractions.

SUMMARY

These cases describe the safety measures taken in preparation for complications from laser lead extractions, which are rare but can cause significant morbidity and mortality. The risk assessment of patient and device characteristics along with assessment of imaging studies, comorbidities, and laboratory work can be critical in preoperative assessment of patient. The preparation enacted to prevent complications or to mitigate loss of time in the event of complications are crucial to a successful program.

CLINICS CARE POINTS

- Patient-related risk factors for superior vena cava injury during transvenous lead extraction include female sex, low body mass index, diabetes mellitus, renal failure, severe left ventricular dysfunction, and anemia.

- The procedure-related risk factors for superior vena cava injury during transvenous lead extraction include presence of superior vena cava occlusion or stenosis and presence of device infection.

- Device-related risk factors for superior vena cava injury during transvenous lead extraction include lead type and duration of implantation and number of leads implanted.

- Preoperative preparation and a multidisciplinary approach to transvenous lead extraction can lead to timely and optimal management of complications including superior vena cava injury.

REFERENCES

1. Perez AA, Woo FW, Tsang DC, et al. Transvenous lead extractions: current approaches and future trends. Arrhythm Electrophysiol Rev 2018;7(3):210–7.

2. Deshmukh A, Patel N, Noseworthy PA, et al. Trends in use and adverse outcomes associated with transvenous lead removal in the United States. Circulation 2015;132(25):2363–71.

3. Wazni O, Epstein LM, Carrillo RG, et al. Lead extraction in the contemporary setting: the LExICon study: an observational retrospective study of consecutive laser lead extractions [published correction appears in J Am Coll Cardiol. 2010 Mar 9;55(10):1055]. J Am Coll Cardiol 2010;55(6):579–86.

4. Arora Y, D'Angelo L, Azarrafiy R, et al. Location of superior vena cava tears in transvenous lead extraction. Ann Thorac Surg 2022;113(4):1165–71.

5. Bashir J, Lee AJ, Philippon F, et al. Predictors of perforation during lead extraction: results of the Canadian lead ExtrAction risk (CLEAR) study. Heart Rhythm 2022;19(7):1097–103.

6. Sood N, Martin DT, Lampert R, et al. Incidence and predictors of perioperative complications with transvenous lead extractions: real-world experience with national cardiovascular data registry. Circ Arrhythm Electrophysiol 2018;11(2):e004768.

7. Jacheć W, Polewczyk A, Polewczyk M, et al. Transvenous lead extraction safety score for risk stratification and proper patient selection for removal procedures using mechanical tools. J Clin Med 2020;9(2):361.

8. Byrd CL, Wilkoff BL, Love CJ, et al. Clinical study of the laser sheath for lead extraction: the total experience in the United States. Pacing Clin Electrophysiol 2002;25(5):804–8.

9. Jacheć W, Polewczyk A, Polewczyk M, et al. Risk factors predicting complications of transvenous lead extraction. BioMed Res Int 2018;2018:8796704.

10. Brunner MP, Cronin EM, Duarte VE, et al. Clinical predictors of adverse patient outcomes in an experience of more than 5000 chronic endovascular pacemaker and defibrillator lead extractions. Heart Rhythm 2014;11(5):799–805.

11. Barakat AF, Wazni OM, Tarakji KG, et al. Transvenous lead extraction in chronic kidney disease and dialysis patients with infected cardiac devices. Circ Arrhythm Electrophysiol 2018;11(1):e005706.

12. Aleong RG, Zipse MM, Tompkins C, et al. Analysis of outcomes in 8304 patients undergoing lead extraction for infection. J Am Heart Assoc 2020;9(7):e011473.

13. Byrd CL, Wilkoff BL, Love CJ, et al. Intravascular extraction of problematic or infected permanent pacemaker leads: 1994-1996. U.S. Extraction Database, MED Institute. Pacing Clin Electrophysiol 1999;22(9):1348–57.

14. Tułecki Ł, Polewczyk A, Jacheć W, et al. Analysis of risk factors for major complications of 1500 transvenous lead extraction procedures with especial attention to tricuspid valve damage. Int J Environ Res Public Health 2021;18(17):9100. Published 2021 Aug 28.

15. Fu HX, Huang XM, Zhong LI, et al. Outcomes and complications of lead removal: can we establish a risk stratification schema for a collaborative and effective approach? [published correction appears in pacing clin electrophysiol. 2016 Feb;39(2):205. Pacing Clin Electrophysiol 2015;38(12):1439–47.

16. Zucchelli G, Di Cori A, Segreti L, et al. Major cardiac and vascular complications after transvenous lead extraction: acute outcome and predictive factors from the ESC-EHRA ELECTRa (European Lead Extraction ConTRolled) registry. Europace 2019;21(5):771–80.

17. Roux JF, Pagé P, Dubuc M, et al. Laser lead extraction: predictors of success and complications. Pacing Clin Electrophysiol 2007;30(2):214–20.

18. Epstein LM, Love CJ, Wilkoff BL, et al. Superior vena cava defibrillator coils make transvenous lead extraction more challenging and riskier. J Am Coll Cardiol 2013;61(9):987–9.

19. Kohut AR, Grammes J, Schulze CM, et al. Percutaneous extraction of ePTFE-coated ICD leads: a single center comparative experience. Pacing Clin Electrophysiol 2013;36(4):444–50.

20. Di Cori A, Bongiorni MG, Zucchelli G, et al. Transvenous extraction performance of expanded polytetrafluoroethylene covered ICD leads in comparison to traditional ICD leads in humans. Pacing Clin Electrophysiol 2010;33(11):1376–81.

21. Segreti L, Di Cori A, Soldati E, et al. Major predictors of fibrous adherences in transvenous implantable cardioverter-defibrillator lead extraction. Heart Rhythm 2014;11(12):2196–201.

22. Svennberg E, Jacobs K, McVeigh E, et al. Computed tomography-guided risk assessment in percutaneous lead extraction. JACC Clin Electrophysiol 2019;5(12):1439–46.

23. Beaser AD, Aziz Z, Besser SA, et al. Characterization of lead adherence using intravascular ultrasound to assess difficulty of transvenous lead extraction. Circ Arrhythm Electrophysiol 2020;13(8):e007726.

24. Patel D, Vatterott P, Piccini J, et al. Prospective evaluation of the correlation between gated cardiac computed tomography detected vascular fibrosis and ease of transvenous lead extraction. Circ Arrhythm Electrophysiol 2022;15(11):e010779.

25. Aboelhassan M, Bontempi L, Cerini M, et al. The role of preoperative venography in predicting the difficulty of a transvenous lead extraction procedure. J Cardiovasc Electrophysiol 2022;33(5):1034–40.

26. Czajkowski M, Jacheć W, Polewczyk A, et al. The influence of lead-related venous obstruction on the

complexity and outcomes of transvenous lead extraction. Int J Environ Res Public Health 2021; 18(18):9634.

27. Wilkoff BL, Love CJ, Byrd CL, et al. Transvenous lead extraction: heart Rhythm Society expert consensus on facilities, training, indications, and patient management: this document was endorsed by the American Heart Association (AHA). Heart Rhythm 2009;6(7):1085–104.

28. Zheng Q, Maytin M, John RM, et al. Transvenous lead extraction during uninterrupted warfarin therapy: feasibility and outcomes. Heart Rhythm 2018; 15(12):1777–81.

29. Vinit S, Vanessa C, Alexander B, et al. Transvenous lead extraction on uninterrupted anticoagulation: a safe approach? Indian Pacing Electrophysiol J 2021;21(4):201–6.

30. Issa ZF, Elayyan MAM. Outcome of transvenous lead extraction in patients on minimally interrupted periprocedural direct oral anticoagulation therapy. J Cardiovasc Electrophysiol 2021;32(10):2722–8.

31. Kusumoto FM, Schoenfeld MH, Wilkoff BL, et al. 2017 HRS expert consensus statement on cardiovascular implantable electronic device lead management and extraction [published correction appears in Heart Rhythm. 2021 Oct;18(10):1814. Heart Rhythm 2017;14(12):e503–51.

32. Goya M, Nagashima M, Hiroshima K, et al. Lead extractions in patients with cardiac implantable electronic device infections: single center experience. J Arrhythm 2016;32(4):308–12.

33. Hussein AA, Wilkoff BL. Transvenous lead extraction of cardiac implantable electronic devices: who, when, how and where? Rev Esp Cardiol 2016;69(1):3–6.

34. Nowosielecka D, Jacheć W, Polewczyk A, et al. Transesophageal echocardiography as a monitoring tool during transvenous lead extraction-does it improve procedure effectiveness? J Clin Med 2020;9(5):1382.

35. Caiati C, Luzzi G, Pollice P, et al. A novel clinical perspective on new masses after lead extraction (ghosts) by means of intracardiac echocardiography. J Clin Med 2020;9(8):2571.

36. Latanich CA, Anderson JA. Shockwave intravascular lithotripsy facilitated transvenous lead extraction. JACC Clin Electrophysiol 2023;9(8 Pt 2):1585–92.

37. Franceschi F, Dubuc M, Deharo JC, et al. Extraction of transvenous leads in the operating room versus electrophysiology laboratory: a comparative study. Heart Rhythm 2011;8(7):1001–5.

38. Sidhu BS, Ayis S, Gould J, et al. Risk stratification of patients undergoing transvenous lead extraction with the ELECTRa Registry Outcome Score (EROS): an ESC EHRA EORP European lead extraction ConTRolled ELECTRa registry analysis. Europace 2021;23(9):1462–71.

39. Kancharla K, Acker NG, Li Z, et al. Efficacy and safety of transvenous lead extraction in the device laboratory and operating room guided by a novel risk stratification scheme. JACC Clin Electrophysiol 2019;5(2):174–82.

40. Bontempi L, Vassanelli F, Cerini M, et al. Predicting the difficulty of a lead extraction procedure: the LED index. J Cardiovasc Med 2014;15(8):668–73.

41. Roberto M, Sicuso R, Manganiello S, et al. Cardiac surgeon and electrophysiologist shoulder-to-shoulder approach: hybrid room, a kingdom for two. A zero mortality transvenous lead extraction single center experience. Int J Cardiol 2019;279:35–9.

42. Kosior J, Jacheć W, Polewczyk A, et al. To grade or not to grade safety requirements for transvenous lead extraction: experience with 2216 procedures. Kardiol Pol 2023;81(3):242–51.

43. Azarrafiy R, Tsang DC, Wilkoff BL, et al. Endovascular occlusion balloon for treatment of superior vena cava tears during transvenous lead extraction: a multiyear analysis and an update to best practice protocol. Circ Arrhythm Electrophysiol 2019;12(8):e007266.

44. Tsang DC, Azarrafiy R, Pecha S, et al. Long-term outcomes of prophylactic placement of an endovascular balloon in the vena cava for high-risk transvenous lead extractions. Heart Rhythm 2017;14(12):1833–8.

Transvenous Lead Extraction in the Left Ventricular Assist Device Patient

Sunil Kapur, MD, Thomas M. Tadros, MD, Melanie Maytin, MD, MSc*

KEYWORDS

- Transvenous lead extraction • Lead management • Left ventricular assist device • Infection
- Implantable cardioverter defibrillator

KEY POINTS

- The population of patients with combined CIEDs and LVADs is increasing dramatically.
- CIED management guidelines are lacking.
- Single-center observational studies suggest that TLE can be performed safely in patients with LVADs.
- Larger, multicenter studies are needed to help guide practitioners in CIED management in the LVAD population.

INTRODUCTION

The population of patients with advanced heart failure continues to increase steadily as does the need for mechanical circulatory support.[1] Between 2500 and 3000 left ventricular assist devices (LVAD) are implanted annually in the United States alone with more than 80% of LVADs implanted in 2022 implanted as destination therapy.[2] Technological device advances promising longer life expectancies combined with the current primary role of LVADs as destination therapy portends an exponential increase in the chronic LVAD population. It is no surprise that the vast majority of patients with LVADs have a cardiovascular implantable electronic device (CIED) given the overlap of indications.[3,4] Moreover, according to current guidelines, implantable cardioverter defibrillator (ICD) therapy is a Class IIa recommendation for patients with an LVAD regardless of whether the device is a bridge to transplant or destination therapy[5] and despite the uncertain role of ICD in the LVAD population.[4,6–11] Thus, the intersection of LVADs and CIEDs is inescapable. Despite this, device management recommendations are limited, and guidelines are lacking.

CLINICAL SCENARIO

A 60-year-old gentleman with nonischemic, dilated cardiomyopathy, status post (s/p) continuous flow (CF) LVAD (HeartMate 3, Abbott, Chicago, Illinois) for cardiogenic shock initially as destination therapy and with subsequent surgical revision of LVAD outflow graft due for outflow graft obstruction presented with ICD lead fracture in a dual-chamber ICD. His arrhythmia and device history are as follows: long-standing atrial fibrillation; aborted sudden cardiac death s/p secondary prevention dual-chamber ICD in 2014; recurrent ventricular arrhythmias (VAs) despite antiarrhythmic therapy with amiodarone; and, following failed ICD shocks in October 2021, defibrillation threshold testing performed yield a defibrillation threshold (DFT) at the maximum output of the device (36J). At this point, mexiletine was added to his antiarrhythmic regimen and amiodarone was

Brigham and Women's Hospital, 75 Francis Street, Boston, MA 02115, USA
* Corresponding author.
E-mail address: mmaytin@bwh.harvard.edu

Card Electrophysiol Clin 16 (2024) 125–132
https://doi.org/10.1016/j.ccep.2023.10.012
1877-9182/24/© 2023 Elsevier Inc. All rights reserved.

discontinued in favor of sotalol in an attempt to chemically lower DFT. He remained relatively quiescent and underwent uncomplicated generator exchange in November 2022. Approximately 3 months later, the patient contacted the clinic for an audible device alarm earlier that morning with remote interrogation demonstrating a bipolar impedance of 1500 Ω. Device interrogation revealed R waves of 3.4 mV, lack of consistent RV capture at maximum output, an ICD lead high voltage impedance of 58 Ω, and an ICD lead pacing impedance of greater than 3000 Ω. Following a multidisciplinary discussion, the decision was made to proceed with ICD transvenous lead extraction (TLE) and replacement. Chronic oral anticoagulation with warfarin was continued uninterrupted perioperatively but with a lower therapeutic goal of 1.8 to 2. International normalized ratio (INR) was 2.2 on the day of TLE. As is our practice, TLE was performed in the operating room under general anesthesia with cardiothoracic surgical backup immediately available. An exchange length super stiff Amplatz guidewire was positioned via the sheath under fluoroscopic guidance to the right internal jugular vein for expedited delivery of a rescue balloon in the event of an superior vena cava (SVC) tear. After opening the CIED pocket and removing the generator, the leads were freed from encapsulating scar tissue to the venous entry point. Using a modified Seldinger technique, the left subclavian vein was accessed with fluoroscopic guidance and a guidewire advanced to the right heart. The active fixation mechanism of the lead was retracted. The lead was cut, and a locking stylet was advanced distally. Using a 16F laser sheath and countertraction, the lead was removed in its entirety. A new ICD lead was implanted while the chronic atrial lead was retained. Hemostasis was achieved with limited electrocautery and absorbable hemostatic powder. The device and leads were placed in an antimicrobial pouch, and the incision was closed in layers. A prophylactic pressure dressing was applied for 7 days, and postprocedure antibiotics were administered for 5 days. Of note, the patient was listed for cardiac transplant in November 2021 and underwent orthotopic heart transplant with complete CIED removal in May 2023 for refractory VAs.

DISCUSSION

VAs and ICD therapies are common after LVAD implantation, occurring with an estimated incidence of 20% to 50%[10,12–17] and 16% to 42%[8,17–21] of patients with LVADs, respectively. Although VAs are thought typically better tolerated among patients with LVADs, they can impair right ventricular function, reduce LVAD flows, and potentiate thrombosis, and are associated with a worse prognosis.[3,11,22,23] However, the benefit of ICD therapy in patients with LVADs is uncertain. Retrospective, observational studies have demonstrated variable benefit of ICD therapy with more recent studies of CF LVAD demonstrating no mortality benefit with ICD therapy.[4,6–10,20,24] Absent a prospective, randomized controlled trial to definitively determine the benefit of ICD therapy in the LVAD population, the decision for defibrillator therapy in patients with LVADs should be individualized with current guidelines recommending ICD implantation in patients with LVADs to treat VAs.[5]

Although the CIED-LVAD population is rapidly expanding, so too are the challenges of CIED management in this patient population—generator exchange, lead malfunction, and infection, to name a few. With advances in medical therapy and LVAD technology, patients with CIED-LVAD are living longer and reaching ICD generator battery depletion. CIED procedures, and, specifically, generator replacements are not without significant risk in this patient population. The observed rate of pocket hematoma ranges from 10% to 19% across several studies.[25–28] This finding is not unexpected given the near universal use of oral anticoagulation and antiplatelet therapy in this patient population as well as the expected platelet dysfunction and acquired von Willebrand factor deficiency. Additionally, generator replacement in patients with CIED-LVAD is associated with a higher rate of infection with reported device infection rates up to 16 times higher.[25–29]

CIED malfunction is common in patients with LVADs, occurring in up to 30% of ICD patients undergoing LVAD implantation.[19,21,28,30–32] Observed types of malfunction include high capture thresholds, ventricular undersensing, lead fracture, and failure to cardiovert. The mechanisms of ICD lead malfunction are incompletely understood. Postulated hypotheses include lead damage; myocardial inflammation, edema, and ischemia; microdislodgement; left ventricular (LV) unloading leading to changes in LV size and septal shift; and alterations in cardiac orientation.[33] Furthermore, management decisions are complicated by the uncertain benefit of ICD therapy on survival and the presumed higher risk associated with TLE in the LVAD population.

Although LVAD infections are a common complication associated with increased mortality,[34–36] less is known about the incidence and outcomes of CIED-LVAD infections. Moreover, there is no consensus as to the best clinical practice. In a retrospective, single-center study of bacteremia in patients with CIED-LVAD, 89% of patients were treated with antibiotics alone. Even though only 10% were treated with surgical management, TLE was associated with a trend toward increased survival.[35] In contrast, other studies have demonstrated increased mortality following CIED infection regardless of successful TLE[37–39] similar to the observed outcomes in non-LVAD populations.[40]

CIED removal is an essential component in the management of CIED-LVAD infection. It has long been accepted that incomplete device removal in CIED infection can result in significant morbidity and mortality.[41–43] More recently, Huang and colleagues observed that TLE alone was curative in patients with CIED infection and prosthetic valves.[44] It is postulated that hardware in the low-pressure venous system is more susceptible to the development of a biofilm than hardware in the high-pressure arterial system such as prosthetic valves and LVADs.

Data surrounding TLE outcomes in patients with LVADs are sparse (**Table 1**). Small, single-center TLE series in patients with LVADs were reported by Krishnamoorthy and colleagues and Riaz and colleagues[38,39] on their experience with TLE in 6 patients each but only Krishnamoorthy and colleagues described the noted procedural characteristics. In this series, the mean implant duration was 5.2 years and two-thirds of the TLE procedures were performed with excimer laser sheath assistance. There were no reported procedural complications but the prognosis of patients after TLE remained poor. Narui and colleagues described their experience with TLE in 11 patients with LVADs as a subgroup analysis of a larger cohort although specific procedural details for the LVAD group are lacking.[45] Black-Maier and colleagues have described the largest single-center experience with TLE in a total of 27 patients with LVADs. Sixty-eight leads with a median implant duration of 5.7 years were removed with 94% complete procedural success and no major complications. All procedures used excimer laser sheaths, 40% of procedures also necessitated mechanical cutting sheath assistance, and 15% required femoral extraction. The majority of patients were managed with chronic suppressive antibiotic therapy.[37] Only one series has included patients with noninfectious indications for TLE. Of 13 patients with LVADs undergoing TLE, the indication for extraction in 3 patients was lead malfunction. The median lead implant duration was 6.3 years, more than three-fourths of patients required extraction sheath assistance, and there were no major complications.[46] The majority of reported studies lack details regarding preprocedural anticoagulation management and postprocedural pocket

care.[35,37,38,45] In the remaining series, oral anticoagulation was interrupted, and bridging with unfractionated heparin was performed in the majority of patients. TLE was performed on uninterrupted warfarin with therapeutic INR (2.2–2.9) in 3 patients. (Maytin M. Safety and Efficacy of Transvenous Lead Extraction in Ventricular Assist Device Patients. In: Unpublished work. 2016).

Current consensus statement guideline recommendations regarding TLE in patients with CIED-LVAD are limited.[47] The only mention of the patient population with CIED-LVAD is a Class I recommendation (level of evidence: consensus—expert opinion) for CIED removal in cases of infection to eliminate a source of potential infection and microbial seeding with a simultaneous recommendation for chronic suppressive antibiotic therapy in those with concomitant LVAD infection. Management decisions for other scenarios in this patient population must be extrapolated.

Although the available limited data suggest that lead extraction can be performed safely in the LVAD population, patients with CIED-LVAD present particular challenges with respect to TLE procedural management. The differences in management begin with preprocedural planning. In addition to the usual multidisciplinary extraction team of cardiothoracic surgeons, cardiac anesthesiologists, and cardiac electrophysiologists, patient management, including the decision to perform TLE, should be expanded to include advanced heart failure cardiologists, infectious disease specialists, anticoagulation management specialists, and mechanical support teams. With almost 1 in 5 patients suffering complications following CIED procedures, special consideration should be given to interventions that may help mitigate these adverse events such as a lower targeted goal INR preprocedure[48,49] or uninterrupted therapeutic oral anticoagulation,[50–52] routine utilization of antimicrobial pouches,[53] and prophylactic pressure dressings.[54] There is a growing body of evidence supporting the safety of TLE on uninterrupted oral anticoagulation.[50–52] This evidence combined the safety of low-intensity warfarin in centrifugal CF LVAD[48,49] argues for uninterrupted therapeutic oral anticoagulation or lower targeted goal INR preprocedure in CIED-LVAD lead extraction procedures. Repeat infection after extraction of infected CIED is unfortunately common.[45] This risk is heightened by the reality that LVAD exchange is infrequently performed in most CIED-LVAD infections. As such, periprocedural antibiotic management and consideration of chronic suppressive antibiotic therapy as well as thoughtful attention to the necessity, timing, and location of CIED reimplant are essential. Moreover,

Table 1
Transvenous lead extraction outcomes in patients with left ventricular assist devices

Study	Study Type	Group Studied	No. Pts	No. Leads	Implant Duration	TLE Tools	Success	Major Complications	LVAD Type	Comments
Schaffer et al,[35] 2023	RO	LVAD-CIED infection	5	NA	NA	NA	NA	NA	NA	Analysis of medical vs surgical management
Black-Maier et al,[37] 2020	RO	LVAD-CIED infection	27	68	5.7 y (median)	Laser 100%[a] Mech. cutting 41% Femoral 15%	94% complete success	None	HVAD 22% HM2 56% HM3 22%	Chronic suppressive antibiotics 83%
Riaz et al,[38] 2014	RO	LVAD-CIED infection	6	NA	NA	NA	NA	NA	HM2 100%	Trial designed to look at CIED infection incidence after LVAD
Krishnamoorthy et al,[39] 2014	RO	LVAD-CIED infection	6	16	5.2 y (mean)	Laser 67% Traction 33%	83% complete success	None	HM2 83% EC 17%	One patient with 1 mo lead implant duration
Narui et al,[45] 2021	RO	Repeat infection after TLE for infection	11	NA	NA	NA	NA	NA	NA	LVAD-CIED infection represents a subgroup
	RO		13	50	NA[c]			None	NA	

			Therapeutic INR in 3 patients
Gosev et al,[46] 2015, Maytin M. Safety and Efficacy of Transvenous Lead Extraction in Ventricular Assist Device Patients. In: Unpublished work. 2016	LVAD-CIED TLE[b]	6.3 y (median)	100% complete success

Abbreviations: CIED, cardiovascular implantable electronic device; EC, extracorporeal pulsatile flow left ventricular assist device; HM2, HeartMate 2; HM3, HeartMate 3; HVAD, HeartWare left ventricular assist device; LVAD, left ventricular assist device; NA, not available; No., number; RO, retrospective observational; TLE, transvenous lead extraction.

[a] 14Fr sheath in 85% and 16Fr sheath in 15% (Spectranetics, Philips, Colorado Springs, Colorado).
[b] Indication: infection 69% and lead malfunction 31%.
[c] Mechanical sheaths used in 77%.

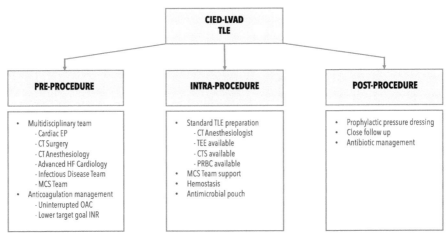

Fig. 1. TLE Considerations in patients with CIED-LVAD. Ensuring favorable outcomes with CIED-LVAD lead extraction requires not only adherence to expected TLE best practice guidelines but also consideration of specific modifiable variables at all stages of the procedure. Preprocedure preparation should include joint decision-making via a multidisciplinary team and consideration of periprocedural oral anticoagulation management. Standard of care guideline-directed steps should be followed in the performance of the procedure. Additionally, the mechanical circulatory support team should be immediately available. Careful attention should be paid to hemostasis during the procedure and an antimicrobial pouch implanted unless contraindicated. Postprocedure considerations include placement of a prophylactic pressure dressing, close follow-up, and consideration of postprocedure antibiotic therapy. CIED, cardiovascular implantable electronic device; CT, cardiothoracic; CTS, cardiothoracic surgeon; EP, electrophysiology; HF, heart failure; INR, international normalized ratio; LVAD, left ventricular assist device; MCS, mechanical circulatory support; OAC, oral anticoagulation; PRBC, packed red blood cell; TEE, transesophageal echocardiography.

in noninfectious TLE indications, it is obvious that assiduous attention to sterile technique and universal utilization of antimicrobial pouches are imperative. To this end, the prevention of pocket hematoma with prophylactic pressure dressing is equally important. Ensuring favorable outcomes with CIED-LVAD lead extraction requires not only adherence to expected TLE best practice guidelines but also consideration of specific modifiable variables (**Fig. 1**).

Finally, recall that the 2017 HRS Guidelines note with Class I indication that careful discussion with the patient needs to be had regarding the risk–benefit ratio of abandonment versus extraction. In our clinical case above, the patient's subclavian vein was patent, the lead was not infected, and there was no issue with overcrowding the venous system. Thus, there was no Class I indication for extraction. We did have the option to abandon the existing lead and add a new lead.

FUTURE DIRECTIONS

This case illustrates many of the multitude of issues that surround CIED lead management in patients with LVADs but perhaps, more importantly, highlights the need for further guidance. Large, prospective studies are needed to understand

the role of CIEDs in patients with newer generation LVADs. Moreover, multicenter reporting of TLE in patients with CIED-LVAD will help formulate guidelines for this patient population.

DISCLOSURE

Dr M. Maytin has received research grants from and is a consultant for Medtronic.

REFERENCES

1. Miller LW, Guglin M. Patient selection for ventricular assist devices: a moving target. J Am Coll Cardiol 2013;61:1209–21.
2. Yuzefpolskaya M, Schroeder SE, Houston BA, et al. The society of thoracic surgeons intermacs 2022 annual report: focus on the 2018 heart transplant allocation system. Ann Thorac Surg 2023;115: 311–27.
3. Berg DD, Vaduganathan M, Upadhyay GA, et al. Cardiac implantable electronic devices in patients with left ventricular assist systems. J Am Coll Cardiol 2018;71:1483–93.
4. Clerkin KJ, Topkara VK, Mancini DM, et al. The role of implantable cardioverter defibrillators in patients bridged to transplantation with a continuous-flow left ventricular assist device: a propensity score

matched analysis. J Heart Lung Transplant 2017;36: 633–9.

5. Al-Khatib SM, Stevenson WG, Ackerman MJ, et al. 2017 AHA/ACC/HRS guideline for management of patients with ventricular arrhythmias and the prevention of sudden cardiac death: a report of the American college of cardiology/American heart association task force on clinical practice guidelines and the heart rhythm society. J Am Coll Cardiol 2018;72:e91–220.

6. Clerkin KJ, Topkara VK, Demmer RT, et al. Implantable cardioverter-defibrillators in patients with a continuous-flow left ventricular assist device: an analysis of the INTERMACS registry. JACC Heart Fail 2017;5:916–26.

7. Younes A, Al-Kindi SG, Alajaji W, et al. Presence of implantable cardioverter-defibrillators and wait-list mortality of patients supported with left ventricular assist devices as bridge to heart transplantation. Int J Cardiol 2017;231:211–5.

8. Lee W, Tay A, Subbiah RN, et al. Impact of implantable cardioverter defibrillators on survival of patients with centrifugal left ventricular assist devices. Pacing Clin Electrophysiol 2015;38:925–33.

9. Enriquez AD, Calenda B, Miller MA, et al. The role of implantable cardioverter-defibrillators in patients with continuous flow left ventricular assist devices. Circ Arrhythm Electrophysiol 2013;6:668–74.

10. Garan AR, Yuzefpolskaya M, Colombo PC, et al. Ventricular arrhythmias and implantable cardioverter-defibrillator therapy in patients with continuous-flow left ventricular assist devices: need for primary prevention? J Am Coll Cardiol 2013;61:2542–50.

11. Gopinathannair R, Cornwell WK, Dukes JW, et al. Device therapy and arrhythmia management in left ventricular assist device recipients: a scientific statement from the American heart association. Circulation 2019;139:e967–89.

12. Raasch H, Jensen BC, Chang PP, et al. Epidemiology, management, and outcomes of sustained ventricular arrhythmias after continuous-flow left ventricular assist device implantation. Am Heart J 2012;164:373–8.

13. Nakahara S, Chien C, Gelow J, et al. Ventricular arrhythmias after left ventricular assist device. Circ Arrhythm Electrophysiol 2013;6:648–54.

14. Ziv O, Dizon J, Thosani A, et al. Effects of left ventricular assist device therapy on ventricular arrhythmias. J Am Coll Cardiol 2005;45:1428–34.

15. Bedi M, Kormos R, Winowich S, et al. Ventricular arrhythmias during left ventricular assist device support. Am J Cardiol 2007;99:1151–3.

16. Andersen M, Videbaek R, Boesgaard S, et al. Incidence of ventricular arrhythmias in patients on long-term support with a continuous-flow assist device (HeartMate II). J Heart Lung Transplant 2009; 28:733 5.

17. Refaat M, Chemaly E, Lebeche D, et al. Ventricular arrhythmias after left ventricular assist device implantation. Pacing Clin Electrophysiol 2008;31: 1246–52.

18. Oswald H, Schultz-Wildelau C, Gardiwal A, et al. Implantable defibrillator therapy for ventricular tachyarrhythmia in left ventricular assist device patients. Eur J Heart Fail 2010;12:593–9.

19. Ambardekar AV, Lowery CM, Allen LA, et al. Effect of left ventricular assist device placement on preexisting implantable cardioverter-defibrillator leads. J Card Fail 2010;16:327–31.

20. Refaat MM, Tanaka T, Kormos RL, et al. Survival benefit of implantable cardioverter-defibrillators in left ventricular assist device-supported heart failure patients. J Card Fail 2012;18:140–5.

21. Pausch J, Mersmann J, Bhadra OD, et al. Prognostic impact of implantable cardioverter defibrillators and associated adverse events in patients with continuous flow left ventricular assist devices. Front Cardiovasc Med 2023;10:1158248.

22. Parikh V, Sauer A, Friedman PA, et al. Management of cardiac implantable electronic devices in the presence of left ventricular assist devices. Heart Rhythm 2018;15:1089–96.

23. Ho G, Braun OO, Adler ED, et al. Management of arrhythmias and cardiac implantable electronic devices in patients with left ventricular assist devices. JACC Clin Electrophysiol 2018;4:847–59.

24. Cantillon DJ, Tarakji KG, Kumbhani DJ, et al. Improved survival among ventricular assist device recipients with a concomitant implantable cardioverter-defibrillator. Heart Rhythm 2010;7:466–71.

25. Eulert-Grehn JJ, Sterner I, Schoenrath F, et al. Defibrillator generator replacements in patients with left ventricular assist device support: the risks of hematoma and infection. J Heart Lung Transplant 2022; 41:810–7.

26. Gilge JL, Sbircea N, Tong MZ, et al. Incidence of cardiac implantable electronic device complications in patients with left ventricular assist devices. JACC Clin Electrophysiol 2021;7:494–501.

27. Black-Maier E, Lewis RK, Loungani R, et al. Cardiovascular implantable electronic device surgery following left ventricular assist device implantation. JACC Clin Electrophysiol 2020;6:1131–9.

28. Ravichandran A, Pothineni NVK, Trivedi JR, et al. Implantable cardioverter-defibrillator-related procedures and associated complications in continuous flow left ventricular assist device recipients: a multicenter experience. Heart Rhythm O2 2021;2:691–7.

29. Burri H. Cardiovascular implantable electronic device procedures in patients with left ventricular assist devices: balancing risks with benefit. JACC Clin Electrophysiol 2020;6:1140–3.

30. Thomas IC, Cork DP, Levy A, et al. ICD lead parameters, performance, and adverse events following

continuous-flow LVAD implantation. Pacing Clin Electrophysiol 2014;37:464–72.

31. Galand V, Leclercq C, Bourenane H, et al. Implantable cardiac defibrillator leads dysfunction after LVAD implantation. Pacing Clin Electrophysiol 2020;43:1309–17.

32. Black-Maier E, Lewis RK, Rehorn M, et al. Implantable cardioverter-defibrillator lead revision following left ventricular assist device implantation. J Cardiovasc Electrophysiol 2020;31:1509–18.

33. Hu YL, Kasirajan V, Tang DG, et al. Prospective evaluation of implantable cardioverter-defibrillator lead function during and after left ventricular assist device implantation. JACC Clin Electrophysiol 2016;2: 343–54.

34. Pagani FD, Miller LW, Russell SD, et al. Extended mechanical circulatory support with a continuous-flow rotary left ventricular assist device. J Am Coll Cardiol 2009;54:312–21.

35. Schaffer AJ, El-Harasis MA, Tinianow A, et al. Clinical outcomes in patients with bacteremia and concomitant left ventricular assist devices and cardiac implantable electronic devices. Am Soc Artif Intern Organs J 2023;69:782–8.

36. O'Horo JC, Abu Saleh OM, Stulak JM, et al. Left ventricular assist device infections: a systematic review. Am Soc Artif Intern Organs J 2018;64:287–94.

37. Black-Maier E, Piccini JP, Bishawi M, et al. Lead extraction for cardiovascular implantable electronic device infection in patients with left ventricular assist devices. JACC Clin Electrophysiol 2020;6:672–80.

38. Riaz T, Nienaber JJ, Baddour LM, et al. Cardiovascular implantable electronic device infections in left ventricular assist device recipients. Pacing Clin Electrophysiol 2014;37:225–30.

39. Krishnamoorthy A, Pokorney SD, Lewis RK, et al. Cardiac implantable electronic device removal in patients with left ventricular assist device associated infections. J Cardiovasc Electrophysiol 2014;25: 1199–205.

40. Maytin M, Jones SO, Epstein LM. Long-term mortality after transvenous lead extraction. Circ Arrhythm Electrophysiol 2012;5:252–7.

41. Gaynor SL, Zierer A, Lawton JS, et al. Laser assistance for extraction of chronically implanted endocardial leads: infectious versus noninfectious indications. Pacing Clin Electrophysiol 2006;29: 1352–8.

42. Le KY, Sohail MR, Friedman PA, et al. Mayo Cardiovascular Infections Study G. Impact of timing of device removal on mortality in patients with

cardiovascular implantable electronic device infections. Heart Rhythm 2011;8:1678–85.

43. Viganego F, O'Donoghue S, Eldadah Z, et al. Effect of early diagnosis and treatment with percutaneous lead extraction on survival in patients with cardiac device infections. Am J Cardiol 2012;109:1466–71.

44. Huang XM, Fu HX, Zhong L, et al. Outcomes of transvenous lead extraction for cardiovascular implantable electronic device infections in patients with prosthetic heart valves. Circ Arrhythm Electrophysiol 2016;9. https://doi.org/10.1161/CIRCEP. 116.004188.

45. Narui R, Nakajima I, Norton C, et al. Risk factors for repeat infection and mortality after extraction of infected cardiovascular implantable electronic devices. JACC Clin Electrophysiol 2021;7:1182–92.

46. Gosev I, Maytin M, Ejiofor JI, et al. Does transvenous lead extraction improve outcomes for ventricular assist device patients? J Heart Lung Transplant 2015;34:S223.

47. Kusumoto FM, Schoenfeld MH, Wilkoff BL, et al. HRS expert consensus statement on cardiovascular implantable electronic device lead management and extraction. Heart Rhythm 2017;14:e503–51.

48. Mehra MR, Uriel N, Naka Y, et al. A fully magnetically levitated left ventricular assist device - final report. N Engl J Med 2019;380:1618–27.

49. Netuka I, Ivak P, Tucanova Z, et al. Evaluation of low-intensity anti-coagulation with a fully magnetically levitated centrifugal-flow circulatory pump-the MAGENTUM 1 study. J Heart Lung Transplant 2018; 37:579–86.

50. Zheng Q, Maytin M, John RM, et al. Transvenous lead extraction during uninterrupted warfarin therapy: feasibility and outcomes. Heart Rhythm 2018; 15:1777–81.

51. Issa ZF, Elayyan MAM. Outcome of transvenous lead extraction in patients on minimally interrupted periprocedural direct oral anticoagulation therapy. J Cardiovasc Electrophysiol 2021;32:2722–8.

52. Vinit S, Vanessa C, Alexander B, et al. Transvenous lead extraction on uninterrupted anticoagulation: a safe approach? Indian Pacing Electrophysiol J 2021;21:201–6.

53. Tarakji KG, Mittal S, Kennergren C, et al. Antibacterial envelope to prevent cardiac implantable device infection. N Engl J Med 2019;380:1895–905.

54. Essebag V, Verma A, Healey JS, et al. Clinically significant pocket hematoma increases long-term risk of device infection: Bruise control infection study. J Am Coll Cardiol 2016;67:1300–8.

Challenge Accepted
Lead Extraction in a Patient with Persistent Left Superior Vena Cava and Right Superior Vena Cava Occlusion

Mutaz Alkalbani, MBBS[a],*, Victoria Luu, BA[b], Aysha Arshad, MD, FHRS[a,b]

KEYWORDS

- Persistent left superior vena cava • Anomalous venous return • Lead extraction

KEY POINTS

- Lead extraction through persistent left superior vena cava (PLSVC) is feasible and safe.
- Due to challenging anatomy, careful planning is essential to improve extraction outcomes in patients with PLSVC.
- Appropriate cardiac imaging prior to the procedure can help in understanding the anatomy and allow risk stratification.
- Indwelling leads, formation of adhesions, and the acute angulation of the coronary sinus into the right ventricle creates a challenge during lead extraction via PLSVC.

Video content accompanies this article at http://www.cardiacep.theclinics.com.

INTRODUCTION

The number of cardiac implantable electronic devices (CIEDs) implanted every year is on the rise globally, especially in the elderly population, with more than 300,000 implanted devices in the United States annually.[1] This is associated with the increased incidence of ischemic heart disease, an aging population, advanced technology, and expanded access to health care.[2,3] At the same time, the incidence of CIED-related infections is on the rise, disproportionately to the increase in the rate of CIED implantation.[4]

Transvenous lead extraction in patients with CIED-related infection is associated with lower mortality.[5] However, despite the current recommendations, the rates of transvenous lead extraction in patients with CIED-related infection are low.[5]

Persistent left superior vena cava (PLSVC) with occluded right superior vena cava (RSVC) is rare and usually found incidentally during CIED leads placement. Implantation of CIED in PLSVC is challenging due to the unusual anatomy. However, previous reports demonstrated the feasibility of the procedure.[6,7] On the other hand, there are limited number of cases in the literature describing transvenous lead extraction via PLSVC. In this case, the authors report the procedural techniques and challenges in leads extraction in a patient with PLSVC and occluded RSVC.

CASE PRESENTATION

A 69-year-old male patient with symptomatic bradycardia and second-degree atrioventricular block type II, presented for elective permanent pacemaker placement in September 2018. During

[a] Inova Schar Heart and Vascular, 3300 Gallows Road, Falls Church, VA 22042, USA; [b] Carient Heart and Vascular, 8100 Ashton Avenue, Suite 200, Manassas, VA 20109, USA
* Corresponding author.
E-mail address: Mutaz.alkalbani@gmail.com
Twitter: @mutazalkalbani (M.A.)

Card Electrophysiol Clin 16 (2024) 133–138
https://doi.org/10.1016/j.ccep.2023.10.013
1877-9182/24/© 2023 Elsevier Inc. All rights reserved.

the procedure, after the left axillary vein was cannulated, it was noted that the wire was tracking lateral and left of the sternum. Contrast injection was given which revealed a huge PLSVC. A 64 cm wire could not be properly advanced to the right atrium despite many attempts; thus, the decision was made to attempt placement via the right side. Next, the venogram demonstrated a patent right subclavian vein leading to a RSVC with a blind pouch (**Fig. 1**). Two 0.035-inch flexible tip wires were then placed from the right subclavian vein into the left subclavian vein and then through the PLSVC to the coronary sinus (CS) and the right atrium (**Fig. 2**). A 7-French × 25 cm OptiSeal Peel-Away sheath was placed over the wire. Several curved stylets were used to advance the lead from the right atrium into the right ventricle through the CS. The lead was then actively fixed into the right ventricular apex. Advancing the right atrial into the right atrial appendage was smoother. Ventricular pacing showed left bundle branch morphology. The sensing and pacing thresholds were checked and were acceptable. Due to underlying atrioventricular nodal disease, note was made of a high percentage of ventricular pacing from the time of the initial pacemaker implantation. Approximately 4 years later in December 2022, the patient presented with progressively worsening exertional dyspnea. A transthoracic echocardiogram demonstrated a reduction in the left ventricular ejection fraction from 55% at baseline to 35%. Pacemaker interrogation demonstrated a ventricular pacing burden of more than 50% with persistent elevation in the right atrial threshold (3 V at 0.5 milliseconds) with excessive battery drainage

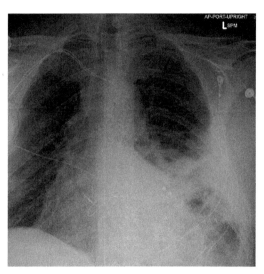

Fig. 2. Pacemaker wires seen crossing to the left side of the chest along via the left superior vena cava into the right atrial appendage and the right ventricle. A left ventricular epicardial lead can also be seen.

and anticipated early depletion. He was diagnosed with pacing-induced cardiomyopathy after excluding ischemia and infiltrative diseases. A recommendation was made to upgrade the dual chamber pacemaker to a cardiac resynchronization pacemaker with the replacement of the right atrial lead. During the extraction procedure with access from right pectoral pocket, manual traction of the atrial lead was not successful. Venogram showed complete occlusion of the right subclavian. After lead preparation, a lead-locking device was then employed. Lead laser extraction system was then utilized, which was calibrated and advanced over the body of the atrial lead into the CS via PLSVC. The lead was then freed into the body of the laser sheath and retracted after delivering several applications of laser energy. Dense adhesions were noted in the right subclavian and subsequently minor adhesions were noted within the PLSVC. A new pacing lead was then advanced to the right atrial appendage via retained access. On venogram it was found that the CS had no lateral branches. A left bundle branch area–pacing lead was introduced and advanced via right subclavian to PLSVC and rotated over to the right ventricular septum. However, this lead was not able to capture adequately due to underlying anatomy and the course of the lead through the PLSVC and CS. After several unsuccessful attempts, the left bundle lead was removed.

The patient was then referred to cardiac surgery for placement of an epicardial left ventricular lead via left thoracotomy which was successfully performed with excellent results. New York Heart

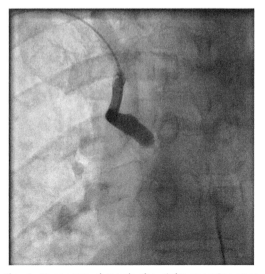

Fig. 1. Venogram through the right superior vena cava demonstrating a blind pouch.

Association class II to III symptoms improved to class I over a few days. After a few weeks following this procedure, the patient presented with a fever. He was found to have cellulitis at the site of the pacemaker pocket with purulent drainage, which led to recommendation for the removal of the complete pacemaker system (Video 1). At the extraction procedure, pus was noted in the pocket, but transesophageal echocardiogram showed no evidence of valve vegetations. A stylet was advanced beyond the pocket and using gentle traction, the right atrial lead was withdrawn without difficulty via the PLSVC. The right ventricular lead was firmly embedded. The lead-locking system was employed. The lead laser extraction system was then calibrated and advanced over the body of the lead using laser cautery into the right atrium through the CS. At this point, the lead itself was freed into the body of the laser sheath and retracted. Given pacemaker dependency, a leadless pacemaker was implanted. This was followed by a staged surgical procedure to remove the left ventricular epicardial lead. The patient had a prolonged hospitalization after extraction and both the thotracotomy site and pacemaker pocket cultures were significant for heavy growth of methicillin-sensitive *Staphylococcus aureus* and *S lugdunensis* and the patient was treated with 6 weeks of nafcillin with recovery.

DISCUSSION
Anatomy of Persistent Left Main Superior Vena Cava

PLSVC is a congenital malformation presenting in approximately 0.3% to 0.5% of the general population.[8] It results when the left anterior cardinal vein fails to obliterate during embryogenesis leading to a persistent left venous system.[9] It begins at the junction of the left subclavian vein and typically drains into the right atrium through the CS. Although, in some cases it drains directly into the left atrium (Cormier and colleagues, 1989[10] and Azizova and colleagues, n.d.). Increased drainage to the right atrium can cause enlargement of the CS, which is the most common indicator of PLSVC existence on echocardiography.[11] The enlargement can also cause structural abnormalities and compression of the conduction pathways leading to conduction abnormalities.[11] Most cases are discovered incidentally during electrophysiologic procedures or placement of central venous catheters. There are anatomic variants associated with PLSVC. In most cases, a right and a left superior venae cavae are present, sometimes with transverse anastomosis.[12] Less often, the caudal RSVC regresses during embryonic stage, resulting

in an absent RSVC with an isolated PLSVC (Jeong and colleagues,[13] 2022). Very rarely, the RSVC partially regresses leading to a pouch that does not connect to the right atrium as in this case.

Lead Implantation via Persistent Left Superior Vena Cava

The approach of implanting CIED leads via PLSVC depends on the anatomy. Different approaches have been described in the literature using the left or the right subclavian veins depending on a transvenous anastomosis. If the patient has dual superior vena cava (SVC), it is easier to implant leads using the right subclavian vein (Beig and colleagues, 2017). The CS drains at an acute angle into the right atrium, which makes it a challenge to advance the leads via the PLSVC into the CS and the right ventricle. Since PLSVC course can be long, a longer lead and sheath might need to be used. Estimating the length of the sheaths can be done by placing the sheath on the body surface under fluoroscopy. Different stylet shapes can be used to overcome the acute angulation, including J-shaped, C-shaped, U-shaped, and pigtail-curved stylets.[9,14] Right ventricular septal stylets and 3D alpha-curved stylets have also been used as described in the literature.[9] A 0.35-inch wire can also be advanced through the PLSVC and CS into the right ventricle, followed by a delivery system over the wire[15] which was also used in our case. The incidence of iatrogenic tricuspid regurgitation from lead placement via PLSVC is unclear. Implanting a right atrial lead via PLSVC and CS is less challenging due to the short distance between the CS orifice and the right atrial appendage and the relatively obtuse angle between the structures.[16] In patients with an indication for cardiac synchronized therapy, implantation of a left ventricular lead is extremely challenging, and in many situations, the procedure is abandoned in favor to an epicardial lead via thoracotomy. The procedure requires a patent CS with adequate branches and collateral connections. Different approaches are described in the literature for successful left ventricular lead placement in patients with challenging anatomy including the use of coronary guidewires, wire externalization, and microcatheters.[17,18] Gul and colleagues described the use of the snaring technique to create a venovenous loop to advance the left ventricular lead.[19] Alternative to biventricular pacing, left bundle branch pacing can be used in patients with cardiomyopathy and a wide QRS interval.[20] Left bundle branch pacing in patients with dual SVC through the right vein has been reported in the literature.[21] However, to the authors' knowledge, there are no cases reported in the literature on successful implantation of a left bundle pacing lead via PLSVC.

Indications for Lead Extraction

The indications for lead extraction are outlined in the 2017 Heart Rhythm Society expert consensus and the 2018 European Heart Rhythm Association expert consensus.[22,23] The most common indication for lead extraction is CIED-related infections including pocket infections, endocarditis, and bacteremia. This is followed by lead dysfunction. However, in certain cases of lead dysfunction, the decision is made to abandon the lead instead of extracting it. Other less common reasons for lead extraction include device upgrade when cardiac resynchronization therapy is indicated or downgrading from a dual to a single chamber system in patients who are in permanent atrial fibrillation. Extractions are also indicated for other lead-related complications such as lead thrombosis, fragment embolism, venous stenosis, or occlusion. Complications of lead extraction procedure are infrequent, although these complications can be tragic requiring urgent surgical intervention. Complications include venous tears or cardiac perforation leading to cardiac tamponade, conduction blocks, pneumothorax, and cardiac arrest.[24] Some of the risk factors associated with higher risk of complications include female gender, longer duration since lead implantation, and number of leads.[24] There are many similarities in the techniques of lead extraction through a PLSVC compared to right-sided systems. However, due to the unusual anatomy, there are special considerations and challenges associated with the procedure. Careful preoperative planning and proper knowledge of the anatomy are important to increase the rates of success and reduce the risk of complications.

Preoperative Planning

The majority of cases reported in the literature of lead extraction from a PLSVC are in the setting of lead infection followed by lead malfunction. Procedures performed in large volume centers with experienced operators are shown to have a higher success rate.[25] Cardiac surgeons and electrophysiologists can be trained to perform the procedure. However, in most cases, cardiac surgery back up should be available for emergent surgical intervention in case needed. The benefits and risks of the procedure should be discussed carefully with the patient and decision makers for mutual decision-making, explaining the other alternatives of the procedure, if an alternative exists.

Preprocedural planning includes performing advanced imaging studies to understand and define the venous anatomy; this includes cardiac computed tomography (CT) scans and cardiac MRI imaging.[26,27] CT scans are also useful in risk stratifying patients to identify features that indicate high complexity such as lead perforation, thrombosis, fractures, or adhesions, and venous stenosis.[28] Other high-risk features include number of leads, duration since leads implantation, and device dependency. Reviewing the implantation procedure is important to understand the challenges in the anatomy during implantation, predict surgical risks of the procedure, and determine the most suitable access site. It also helps to identify and prepare the right instruments that are needed to perform the procedure.

Procedural Techniques

Due to the limited number of cases, there are no standard procedural techniques for lead extraction in patients with PLSVC. Several techniques have been reported, including manual traction, which is usually successful in case of leads that are recently implanted. If manual traction is not successful, standard nonpowered tools such as locking stylets and mechanical dissection sheaths are used.[29] For imbedded leads, powered extraction tools such as laser devices and rotational sheaths are utilized to assist in the lead extraction.[30] Video-assisted thoracoscopy can also be used to monitor the SVC during the procedure.

Complications and Challenges

One of the major challenges of the procedure is overcoming the acute angulation of the PLSVC into the right ventricle through the CS. Lead extraction becomes more challenging when fibrotic adhesions build up around the steep angles. Akhtar and colleagues described the role of rotational tools that provide the flexibility and plasticity to advance through the acute angle, maintaining their ability to dissect through the veins.[30] Compromised lead integrity has also been reported during extraction, during which a femoral intravascular retrieval set was used to extract the lead with a steerable femoral bioptome and a snare.[31] Trenson and colleagues described the use of internal transjugular approach for indwelling leads.[29] As PLSVC connects to the CS posteriorly, fibrotic adhesions at the ostium of the CS can increase the risk of CS tear leading to cardiac tamponade and heart dislocation.[32] Emergent surgical intervention in case of PLSVC tear can be more complicated compared to an RSVC tear given the unusual anatomy of the vessel within the chest cavity.[33] Hence comes the importance of adequate imaging prior to the procedure in order to have a better understanding of the anatomy.

Outcomes

Most cases reported in the literature demonstrated the feasibility and safety of lead extraction through a PLSVC with good outcomes after 12 months. Reimplantation of new leads through the PLSVC after extraction is also possible. Due to the limited number of cases in the literature, there are no sufficient data to compare rates of success or complications compared to traditional lead extraction.

SUMMARY

PLSVC is relatively uncommon. Lead extraction through PLSVC is feasible. However, careful planning should take place prior to the procedure to increase the success rate and reduce the risk of complications. Planning includes preoperative imaging, multidisciplinary team discussion including cardiac surgeons and electrophysiologists, and engaging patients and families in mutual decision-making. Due to unusual anatomy, the procedure carries challenges that might require special tools. More studies are needed to understand the rates of complications and long-term outcomes in patients after PLSVC lead extraction.

ETHICS

The patient provided the consent to share clinical information for publication. No personal identifiers were used. The Inova Health System Institutional Review Board determined that the proposed case report under the number INOVA-2023 to 53 concerning 3 or less patients does not constitute human subjects research as defined by US Department of Health and Human Services and/or US Food and Drug Administration regulations and approval is not required.

DISCLOSURE

The authors have nothing to disclose.

SUPPLEMENTARY DATA

Supplementary data related to this article can be found online at https://doi.org/10.1016/j.ccep.2023.10.013

REFERENCES

1. Greenspon AJ, Patel JD, Lau E, et al. Trends in permanent pacemaker implantation in the United States from 1993 to 2009: increasing complexity of patients and procedures. J Am Coll Cardiol 2012;60(16):1540–5.
2. Bradshaw PJ, Stobie P, Knuiman MW, et al. Trends in the incidence and prevalence of cardiac pacemaker insertions in an ageing population. Open Heart 2014. https://doi.org/10.1136/openhrt-2014.
3. Mond HG, Proclemer A. The 11th world survey of cardiac pacing and implantable cardioverter-defibrillators: calendar year 2009–A world society of arrhythmia's project. Pacing Clin Electrophysiol 2011;34(8):1013–27.
4. Sohail MR, Eby EL, Ryan MP, et al. Incidence, treatment intensity, and incremental annual expenditures for patients experiencing a cardiac implantable electronic device infection: evidence from a large US payer database 1-year post implantation. Circ Arrhythm Electrophysiol 2016;9(8). https://doi.org/10.1161/CIRCEP.116.003929/FORMAT/EPUB.
5. Sciria CT, Kogan EV, Mandler AG, et al. Low utilization of lead extraction among patients with infective endocarditis and implanted cardiac electronic devices. J Am Coll Cardiol 2023;81(17):1714–25.
6. Mazzone P, Guarracini F, Radinovic A, et al. Single chamber pacemaker implantation in a patient with persistent left superior vena cava and right superior vena cava occlusion: a technical challenge solved with a particular right ventricular lead. Int Cardiovasc Res J 2015;9(3):180–2.
7. Guenther M, Kolschmann S, Rauwolf TP, et al. Implantable cardioverter defibrillator lead implantation in patients with a persistent left superior vena cava—feasibility, chances, and limitations: representative cases in adults. EP Europace 2013;15(2):273–7.
8. Tyrak KW, Hołda J, Hołda MK, et al. AFRICA e1 Case report persistent left superior vena cava. Cardiovascular J Africa 2017;28(3):1–4. https://doi.org/10.5830/CVJA-2016-084.
9. Beig JR, Dar MI, Tramboo NA, et al. An innovation in pacemaker lead implantation via persistent left superior vena cava: the "3D alpha curve" stylet. Pacing Clin Electrophysiol 2017;40(9):1042–4.
10. Cormier MG, Yedlicka JW, Gray RJ, et al. Congenital anomalies of the superior vena cava: a CT study. Semin Roentgenol 1989;24(2):77–83.
11. Azizova A, Onder O, Arslan S, et al. Persistent left superior vena cava: clinical importance and differential diagnoses. Insights Imaging 2020. https://doi.org/10.1186/s13244-020-00906-2.
12. Rizkallah J, Burgess J, Kuriachan V. Absent right and persistent left superior vena cava: troubleshooting during a challenging pacemaker implant: a case report. BMC Res Notes 2014;7(1). https://doi.org/10.1186/1756-0500-7-462.
13. Jeong ER, Kang EJ, Jeun JH. Pictorial essay: understanding of persistent left superior vena cava and its

differential diagnosis. J Korean Soc Radiol 2022; 83(4):846–60.

14. Li T, Xu Q, Liao HT, et al. Transvenous dual-chamber pacemaker implantation in patients with persistent left superior vena cava. BMC Cardiovasc Disord 2019;19(1):1–6.

15. Kanjwal K, Soos M, Gonzalez-Morales D, et al. Case report persistent left superior vena cava and absent right superior vena cava with left subclavian vein stenosis: technical challenges with pacemaker implantation. Case Rep Cardiol 2019. https://doi.org/10.1155/2019/7271591.

16. Sánchez-Quintana D, Doblado-Calatrava M, Cabrera JA, et al. Anatomical basis for the cardiac interventional electrophysiologist. Biomed Res Int 2015. https://doi.org/10.1155/2015/547364.

17. Liu YH, Lai LP, Lin JL. Using multiple buddy wires to facilitate left ventricular lead advancement in cardiac resynchronization therapy. J Intervent Card Electrophysiol 2007;18(3):239–41.

18. Furniss GO, Liang M, Jimenez A, et al. Wire externalisation for left ventricular lead placement in cardiac Resynchronisation therapy: a step-by-step guide. Heart Lung Circ 2015;24(11):1094–103.

19. Gul EE, Ali IA, Haseeb YB, et al. Retrograde snaring for left ventricular lead placement in the presence of a persistent left superior vena cavaonline) CC BY 4.0 license. J Innov Cardiac Rhythm Manage 2023; 14(1):5322–4.

20. Pugazhendhi Vijayaraman M, Parikshit S, Sharma MM, et al. Comparison of left bundle branch area pacing and biventricular pacing in candidates for resynchronization therapy. J Am Coll Cardiol 2023. https://doi.org/10.1016/J.JACC.2023.05.006.

21. Prolič Kalinšek T, Žižek D. Right-sided approach to left bundle branch area pacing combined with atrioventricular node ablation in a patient with persistent left superior vena cava and left bundle branch block: a case report. BMC Cardiovasc Disord 2022;22(1). https://doi.org/10.1186/S12872-022-02914-0.

22. Bongiorni MG, Burri H, Deharo JC, et al. EHRA expert consensus statement on lead extraction: recommendations on definitions, endpoints, research trial design, and data collection requirements for clinical scientific studies and registries: endorsed by APHRS/HRS/LAHRS. EP Europace 2018;20(7): 1217.

23. Kusumoto FM, Schoenfeld MH, Wilkoff BL, et al. HRS expert consensus statement on cardiovascular implantable electronic device lead management and extraction. Heart Rhythm 2017;14(12):e503–51.

24. Sood N, Martin DT, Lampert R, et al. Incidence and predictors of perioperative complications with transvenous lead extractions: Real-world experience with National cardiovascular data Registry. Circ Arrhythm Electrophysiol 2018;11(2). https://doi.org/10.1161/CIRCEP.116.004768/-/DC1.

25. Di Monaco A, Pelargonio G, Narducci ML, et al. Safety of transvenous lead extraction according to centre volume: a systematic review and meta-analysis. EP Europace 2014;16(10):1496–507.

26. Sohal M, Ma YL, Rinaldi CA. Laser extraction of a defibrillator lead from a persistent left superior vena cava. EP Europace 2013;15(8):1174.

27. Azizova A, Onder O, Arslan S, et al. Persistent left superior vena cava: clinical importance and differential diagnoses. Insights Imaging 2020. https://doi.org/10.1186/s13244-020-00906-2.

28. Svennberg E, Jacobs K, Mcveigh E, et al. Computed tomography-guided risk assessment in percutaneous lead extraction. JACC Clin Electrophysiol 2019. https://doi.org/10.1016/j.jacep.2019.09.007.

29. Trenson S, Doering M, Hindricks G, et al. Transvenous lead extraction in a patient with persistent left superior vena cava. HeartRhythm Case Rep 2020. https://doi.org/10.1016/j.hrcr.2020.11.025.

30. Akhtar Z, Sohal M, Starck CT, et al. Persistent left superior vena cava transvenous lead extraction: a European experience. J Cardiovasc Electrophysiol 2022;33(1):102–8.

31. Tanawuttiwat T, Brinker J, Rickard J. Left persistent superior vena cava lead extraction using a femoral approach. Europace 2016;18(2):252.

32. Bontempi L, Tempio D, Vito R De, et al. Unexpected challenging case of coronary sinus lead extraction. World J Clin Cases 2017;5(2):46.

33. Akhtar Z, Sohal M, Starck CT, et al. Persistent left superior vena cava transvenous lead extraction: a European experience. J Cardiovasc Electrophysiol 2022;33(1):102–8.

Lead Extraction and Baffle Stenting in a Patient with Transposition of the Great Arteries

Rady Ho, MD[a],*, Nilay Patel, MD[b], Rahul Sakhuja, MD[b],
Ignacio Inglessis-Azuaje, MD[b], Theofanie Mela, MD[b]

KEYWORDS

- Dextro-transposition of the great arteries • Mustard procedure • SVC stent • Baffle stent
- Laser lead extraction • Mechanical rotator sheath

KEY POINTS

- Patient Profile: A 42-year-old male with dextro-transposition of the great arteries (D-TGA) after Mustard repair and sick sinus syndrome, treated with a dual-chamber pacemaker implant.
- Complex Treatment: Developed symptomatic superior vena cava (SVC) baffle stenosis and underwent a combined procedure involving pacemaker extraction and SVC baffle stenting.
- Efficacy Demonstrated: The case showcases the successful outcome of the combined approach in treating SVC baffle stenosis in the presence of cardiac implantable devices.
- Comprehensive Insight: Provides insights into the intricacies of D-TGA, its surgical history, and long-term complications associated with atrial switch procedures.
- Clinical Complexity: Highlights the challenges and considerations involved in managing complex cardiac conditions and the importance of tailored treatment strategies.

INTRODUCTION

Dextro-transposition of the great arteries (D-TGA) is a type of cyanotic congenital heart disease characterized by a reversed position of the aorta and pulmonary artery. The Mustard atrial switch procedure is a surgical intervention employed for the management of the D-TGA. Although the Mustard procedure demonstrates excellent clinical outcomes during the first 2 decadoo of life, important enduring consequences such as superior vena cava (SVC) baffle stenosis can arise. When SVC baffle stenosis occurs in the presence of a pacemaker, a unique management challenge arises. This case report presents a patient with D-TGA and SVC baffle stenosis successfully treated with a combined approach of pacemaker extraction and subsequent SVC baffle stenting.

CASE REPORT

We present a case of a 42-year-old male with a history of D-TGA status post Mustard repair at the age of 8 months with a systemic right ventricle, sick sinus syndrome status post dual-chamber pacemaker implant in 2013, and right bundle branch block who was referred to our institution for management of SVC baffle stenosis. Until late 2019, he was in his normal state of health, but he experienced acute onset reduced exercise tolerance and exertional dyspnea. He was having difficulty carrying out his job and completing his routine 45-minute bike ride between home and work. As result, he underwent extensive cardiac work-up. Coronary angiogram revealed normal epicardial coronary arteries. Transthoracic echocardiogram revealed a new severe right systolic ventricular failure. Computed tomography (CT) chest showed severe focal stenosis of the

[a] Lehigh Valley Heart and Vascular Institute, 1250 South Cedar Crest Boulevard, Allentown, PA 18103, USA;
[b] Corrigan Minehan Heart Center, Massachusetts General Hospital, 55 Fruit Street, Boston, MA 02114, USA
* Corresponding author. 1250 South Cedar Crest Boulevard, #300, Allentown, PA 18103.
E-mail address: rady.ho@lvhn.org

Card Electrophysiol Clin 16 (2024) 139–142
https://doi.org/10.1016/j.ccep.2023.10.003

cardiacEP.theclinics.com

SVC baffle (**Fig. 1**). The etiology of his symptoms and new-onset systolic ventricular failure were thought to be secondary to SVC baffle stenosis. His case was reviewed during a multidisciplinary team meeting consisting of adult congenital cardiologist, cardiovascular surgeons, interventional cardiologists, and electrophysiologists. Due to the challenging anatomy and the proximity of the pacemaker leads to the stenotic area, it was determined that pacemaker leads extraction would be necessary to facilitate SVC baffle stenting. Transvenous lead extraction was performed by the electrophysiology team prior to SVC baffle stenting by interventional cardiology.

Transvenous Lead Extraction

The procedure was performed under general anesthesia in a hybrid operating room with cardiac thoracic surgery backup. His pacemaker was interrogated prior to the procedure, confirming that the patient was not pacemaker dependent. The extraction was guided by fluoroscopy and transesophageal echocardiography. Following insertion of a locking stylet, 0-Ethibond sutures were tied around the insulation of both atrial and ventricular leads to provide additional traction. Despite using laser energy with a Laser sheath, advancing it across the baffle proved to be challenging. Therefore, the laser sheath was exchanged for a mechanical rotating cutting sheath. With the mechanical sheath, the authors were able to advance over the atrial lead through the SVC baffle into the left atrium (LA), and the lead was extracted without resistance. Similarly, the ventricular lead was extracted via the mechanical cutting sheath. Following successful lead extraction, a guidewire was advanced through the SVC and IVC baffles to retain venous access.

Baffle Stenting

Following pacemaker leads extraction, an SVC angiogram showed near total occlusion of the

SVC baffle (**Fig. 2**). First, the stenosis was predilated with balloon angioplasty (**Fig. 3**). After dilatation, the stent was successfully placed around the stenosis(**Fig. 4**). Repeat SVC angiogram at the end of the case showed restoration of venous flow through the SVC baffle (**Fig. 5**).

Pacemaker Implantation

After successful angioplasty and stenting, a dual-chamber pacemaker was inserted in a conventional fashion (**Fig. 6**).

DISCUSSION

Adult congenital heart disease is rapidly growing, and TGA accounts for 7% to 9%[1] of cases. TGA is a type of congenital heart disease characterized by ventriculoarterial discordance. D-TGA is a specific type of TGA in which the aorta originates from the morphologic right ventricle (RV), and the pulmonary artery originates from the morphologic left ventricle (LV).[2] This defect usually is accompanied by an atrial septal defect (ASD), a ventricular septal defect (VSD), or patent ductus arteriosus to allow mixing of oxygenated and de-oxygenated blood earlier on in life. However, surgical repair is almost always necessary early in life for the survival of patients with D-TGA. Atrial switch procedures, such as Senning and Mustard, were the treatment of choice historically. They involve creating SVC and IVC baffles to direct the venous return to the contralateral atrioventricular valve and ventricle. Atrial switch procedure provides excellent clinical result with 40 years survival rate between 60% and 75%.[3]

However, despite the excellent survival rate, long-term complications such as arrhythmia, baffle stenosis, and right ventricular failure are well-recognized.[4] Baffle leak and stenosis are common complications with a prevalence from 10% to 36%.[5] Although it can be asymptomatic, baffle stenosis can lead to hemodynamic overload and heart failure as seen in our patient. In cases of symptomatic baffle stenosis, percutaneous baffle

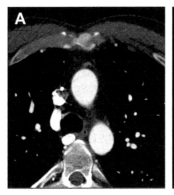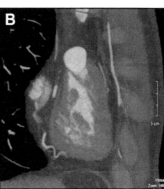

Fig. 1. Pre-operative chest computed tomography (CT) scan showed severe focal stenosis of the superior vena cava (SVC) baffle. (*A*) CT axial view. (*B*) CT sagittal view.

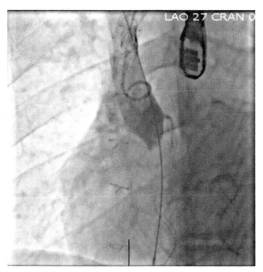

Fig. 2. Following successful pacemaker leads extraction, an SVC baffle venogram showed total occlusion of the SVC baffle.

stenting is the preferred therapeutic intervention over surgical revision when feasible.[6–8]

Due to the elevated risk of sinus node dysfunction, arrhythmia, and sudden death, cardiac implantable devices, including pacemakers and defibrillators, are prevalent in this population, with an incidence of 2% to 15%.[9] Device extraction is often required for various reasons, including device revision, infection, and venous obstruction. While there has been no large randomized trial to date, accumulating evidence supports the safety and effectiveness of transvenous device extraction.[10–12]

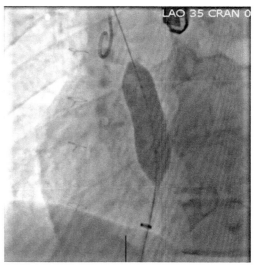

Fig. 4. Deployment of SVC baffle stent following balloon angioplasty.

When SVC baffle stenosis occurs in the presence of cardiac implantable devices, a unique management challenge arises. Management of these patients should involve a multidisplinary team consisting of electrophysiologists and interventional cardiologists. Patients often require concomitant transvenous lead extraction, baffle stenting, and device reimplantation. A combined approach of transvenous lead extraction and baffle stenting appears safe and feasible in D-TGA patients, as supported by previous studies.[13]

In this case report, the authors present a 42-year-old male with a history of D-TGA status

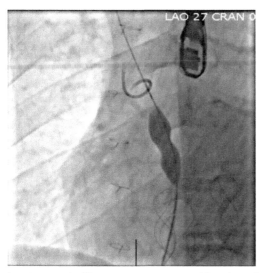

Fig. 3. SVC baffle stenosis was pre-dilated with balloon angioplasty prior to stent deployment.

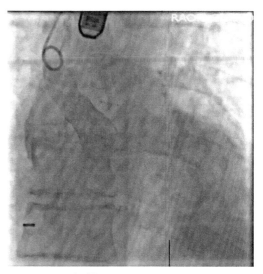

Fig. 5. An SVC baffle venogram showed restoration of blood flow through SVC baffle after stenting.

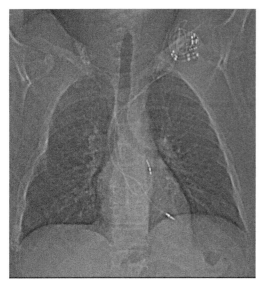

Fig. 6. Chest radiograph showed pacemaker leads position following pacemaker reimplantation.

post Mustard repair and dual-chamber pacemaker who developed SVC baffle stenosis and systemic ventricular failure. The etiology of his ventricular failure was thought to be secondary to baffle stenosis after evaluation ruled out other causes. He subsequently underwent a combined transvenous lead extraction, baffle stenting, and pacemaker reimplantation without complications. This case highlights a few important points. First, transvenous lead extraction often requires both laser and mechanical rotator sheaths. Secondly, it further supports the safety and effectiveness of a combined approach in D-TGA patients.

FUNDING

No funding

CLINICS CARE POINTS

- Baffle stenosis is one of potential complications following the atrial switch procedure.
- Percutaneous baffle stenting is the preferred therapeutic intervention over surgical revision for the treatment of symptomatic baffle stenosis.
- Symptomatic baffle stenosis in the presence of cardiac implantable devices can be safely and effectively treated with a combined transvenous lead extraction and percutaneous baffle stenting.

DISCLOSURE

The authors have no conflict to disclose.

REFERENCES

1. Ávila P, Mercier L-A, Dore A, et al. Adult congenital heart disease: a growing epidemic. Can J Cardiol 2014;30:S410–9.
2. Warnes CA. Transposition of the great arteries. Circulation 2006;114:2699–709.
3. Gelatt M, Hamilton RM, McCrindle BW, et al. Arrhythmia and mortality after the Mustard procedure: a 30-year single-center experience. J Am Coll Cardiol 1997;29:194–201.
4. Cuypers JA, Eindhoven JA, Maarten AS, et al. Eur Heart J 2014;25:1666–74.
5. Khairy P, Landzberg MJ, Lambert J, et al. Long-term outcomes after the atrial switch for surgical correction of transposition: a meta-analysis comparing the Mustard and Senning procedures. Cardiol Young 2004;14:284.
6. Tzifa A, Marshall AC, McElhinney DB, et al. Endovascular treatment for superior vena cava occlusion or obstruction in a pediatric and young adult population: a 22-year experience. J Am Coll Cardiol 2007;49:1003–9.
7. Hill KD, Fleming G, Curt Fudge J, et al. Percutaneous interventions in high-risk patients following Mustard repair of transposition of the great arteries. Cathet Cardiovasc Interv 2012;80:905–14.
8. Baumgartner H, De Backer J, Babu-Narayan B, et al. 2020 ESC Guidelines for the management of adult congenital heart disease. Eur Heart J 2022; 42:563–645.
9. Kammeraad J, Deurzen C, Sreeram N, et al. Predictor of sudden death after mustard or senning repair for transposition of the great arteries. J Am Cool Cardiol 2004;44:1095–102.
10. Cooper JM, Stephenson EA, Berul CI, et al. Implantable cardioverter defibrillator lead complications and laser extraction in children and young adults with congenital heart disease: implications for implantation and management. J Cardiovasc Electrophysiol 2003;14:344–9.
11. McCanta AC, Kong MH, Carboni MP, et al. Laser lead extraction in congenital heart disease: a case controlled study: laser Extraction in CHD. Pacing Clin Electrophysiol 2013;36:372–80.
12. Khairy P, Roux J-F, Dubuc M, et al. Laser lead extraction in adult congenital heart disease. J Cardiovasc Electrophysiol 2007;18:507–11.
13. Laredo M, Waldman V, Chaix MA, et al. Lead extraction with baffle stenting in adults with transposition of the great arteries. JACC Clin Electrophysiol 2019;5: 671–80.

Open Chest Approach Lead Extraction in a Patient with a Large Vegetation

The Importance of Multidisciplinary Approach, Advanced Imaging, and Procedural Planning

Anne-Sophie Lacharite-Roberge, MD[a],*, Kavisha Patel, MD[a],
Yang Yang, MD[a], Ulrika Birgersdotter-Green, MD[a], Travis L. Pollema, DO[b]

KEYWORDS

• Lead extraction • Device infection • Open chest lead extraction • Pacemaker
• Implantable cardiac defibrillator • Vegetation • Endocarditis

KEY POINTS

- Although percutaneous techniques have evolved as the preferred lead and device extraction methods, an open chest approach remains the safest method in some clinical scenarios; presence of a large mass on the leads, prior failed extraction, or presence of a patent foramen ovale increase the risk of embolization.
- The use of vacuum-assisted thrombectomy and debulking systems has been described as an effective technique to reduce the size of a mass to achieve percutaneous extraction in patients who are poor surgical candidates.
- A multidisciplinary approach and prompt referral to an experienced center is crucial in the care of patients with device infection being considered for extraction.

 Video content accompanies this article at http://www.cardiacep.theclinics.com.

INTRODUCTION

It is estimated that each year, approximately 1.7 million cardiac implantable electronic devices (CIEDs) are implanted worldwide.[1] Device-related infections, which occur at a rate of 1% to 2%, remain a serious complication associated with high mortality and morbidity.[2,3] Because implantation rates increase with an aging population and broader clinical indications for CIEDs, clinicians must recognize complications associated with CIEDs and understand the need for prompt referral to an experienced device extraction center when a diagnosis of CIED infection is suspected.

Complete device and lead removal is the recommended treatment for the successful eradication of CIED infection, and the decision to proceed with a percutaneous or open chest approach is a crucial step in patient evaluation.[4] Although percutaneous lead extraction has evolved as the preferred method in the last 3 decades, it is not suitable for every case.[5] The chosen technique

[a] Division of Cardiology, Section of Electrophysiology, University of California San Diego, 9452 Medical Center Drive, La Jolla, CA 92037, USA; [b] Division of Cardiovascular and Thoracic Surgery, University of California San Diego, 9452 Medical Center Drive, La Jolla, CA 92037, USA
* Corresponding author.
E-mail address: alachariteroberge@health.ucsd.edu

Card Electrophysiol Clin 16 (2024) 143–147
https://doi.org/10.1016/j.ccep.2023.10.014

depends on several patient-centered factors including the need for cardiac surgery regardless of the need for extraction, prohibitive risk factors for percutaneous approach, failed prior extraction, or the presence of large masses (vegetation or thrombus >2.5 cm) on cardiac imaging.[6]

We report a complex case of CIED infection, bacteremia, and large lead vegetation where elective open chest extraction was deemed a safer option after comprehensive preprocedural workup including transesophageal echocardiogram (TEE) and computed tomography (CT) lead extraction protocol were completed.

HISTORY

A 55-year-old woman with a past medical history of hypertension, atrial fibrillation ablation, and complete atrioventricular block with a dual-chamber pacemaker placement in 2009 and generator change in 2013 was transferred to our institution for further management of tricuspid valve endocarditis, concern for device infection, subarachnoid hemorrhage, and severe thrombocytopenia. At the time of presentation at an outside institution, the patient reported developing fevers, chills, and generalized malaise while vacationing in another country. Initial workup included a transthoracic echocardiogram (TTE) showing a 7 cm vegetation on the right ventricular pacemaker lead, in addition to multiple smaller sized vegetations affecting the tricuspid valve. Blood cultures were positive for *Lactobacillus* Jensenii. She was initially treated with vancomycin and imipenem, with subsequent narrowing to penicillin after negative blood cultures were obtained for 5 days. Other notable positive studies and results during the patient's initial workup were a platelet count of 5000/mm^3, a subarachnoid hemorrhage in the right frontal lobe discovered on head CT, and a multisegmental pulmonary embolus on CT angiography of the chest. She arrived at our institution in stable condition.

Following her transfer, the patient underwent a CT angiography lead extraction protocol. This confirmed the presence of a large vegetation associated with the right ventricular pacemaker lead, straddling the tricuspid valve plane approximately 3.2 × 1.8 × 2.2 cm in size, and prolapsing across the valve through the cardiac cycle (**Fig. 1**A). Pulmonary embolic disease/septic emboli were redemonstrated in the right middle lobe and likely in the right and left lobes, with evolving pulmonary infarcts. TEE was performed, and it revealed severe tricuspid regurgitation, a flail tricuspid valve, and mobile vegetations on its septal leaflet. There was redemonstration of a large mass/vegetation on the right ventricular

pacing wire, and the study was also significant for the presence of a moderate-sized patent foramen ovale (PFO; **Fig. 1**B). Device interrogation revealed 100% right ventricular pacing burden and 18% atrial pacing burden with stable lead parameters and function. The patient underwent an extensive workup for thrombocytopenia, including a bone marrow biopsy. There were likely multiple contributing causes to the patient's low platelet count, including active infection, treatment with multiple antibiotics, low-grade disseminated intravascular coagulation, and possibly a primary bone marrow process given dysplasia discovered on bone marrow biopsy. Infectious diseases, hematology, neurosurgery, cardiothoracic surgery, and cardiac electrophysiology were consulted to assist in the management of this complex patient.

The initial discussion for the management of the patient's device infection was percutaneous extraction with the use of an aspiration thrombectomy device to avoid sternotomy and cardiopulmonary bypass, which would require moderate dose heparinization. This was deemed high risk in the setting of severe thrombocytopenia and subarachnoid hemorrhage. However, the presence of a moderate-sized PFO on TEE precluded a percutaneous approach due to the risk of embolization of material across the interatrial septum. The decision was therefore made to wait 2 weeks and then proceed with open chest approach lead extraction, placement of a dual-chamber epicardial pacemaker system, tricuspid valve repair, and PFO closure on cardiopulmonary bypass. Platelet goal was set at 200,000/mm^3 and before discharge, hematology recommended the administration of romiplostim for management of thrombocytopenia. The patient also underwent peripherally inserted central catheter line placement and was discharged home with daily intravenous penicillin until surgery.

OPERATIVE COURSE

The patient was taken to the operating room in stable condition on the day of surgery. After induction of general anesthesia, the patient was placed on cardiopulmonary bypass. The heart was fibrillated with external fibrillating cables and the right atrium was opened. PFO closure was performed and the heart was allowed to regain normal sinus rhythm. The pacemaker leads were identified and removed under direct visualization. As suspected, a large mass was present on the right ventricular lead (**Fig. 2**A). All vegetative material was removed and debrided (Video 1). The leads were placed under traction in the superior vena cava and amputated. The tricuspid valve was then carefully inspected, and although the leaflets were thickened, there

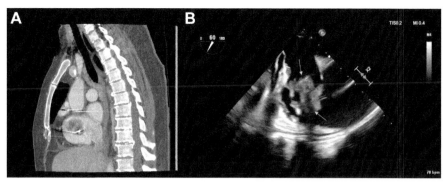

Fig. 1. (*A*) CT lead extraction protocol in the sagittal view showing a large mass (*yellow arrow*) associated with the pacemaker lead. (*B*) Transesophageal echocardiogram demonstrating a large mass across the tricuspid valve (*yellow arrows*).

was no rupture of the chordae or leaflet perforation. There was severe tricuspid regurgitation specifically at the anteroseptal and posteroseptal commissures. Commissuroplasty of the leaflets was performed and testing of the valve revealed near complete resolution of the regurgitation.

Following successful weaning from cardiopulmonary bypass, the pacemaker pocket was opened, and the pulse generator was removed, in addition to the remainder of the leads by gentle traction (**Fig. 2**B). An epicardial dual-chamber pacemaker was placed before chest closure.

The patient had no immediate complication following the surgery and did not require any inotropic or vasopressor support. Before discharge, antibiotics were transitioned to amoxicillin 1 g 3 times a day for 2 additional weeks. About the patient's diagnosis of thrombocytopenia, her platelet count fully recovered, favoring active infection as the most likely cause.

DISCUSSION

We present a case of a patient with CIED infection, bacteremia, large lead vegetation and PFO

requiring open chest approach lead extraction. As recommended by the 2017 Heart Rhythm Society consensus statement on lead management, open surgical techniques are favored when preoperative imaging reveals large lead masses greater than 2.5 cm, in order to prevent embolization. Several case reports and case series have shown that although percutaneous lead extraction is feasible in the presence of large masses, pulmonary embolization is almost inevitable.[7] Another technique described in the literature to achieve percutaneous lead extraction in patients who are poor candidates for open technique is the use of vacuum-assisted thrombectomy and debulking systems, followed by percutaneous device removal.[8–11] In a case series of 8 patients by Godara and colleagues, there was no perioperative embolization events, and all but 1 patient met the desired endpoint of greater than 50% reduction in vegetation size using the AngioVac system (Angiodynamics/Vortex medical Inc, Marlborough, MA, USA).[11]

Our case was unique as the preoperative imaging and testing revealed a moderate-sized PFO, which precluded the use of any percutaneous

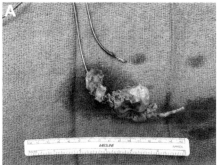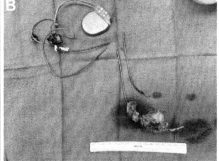

Fig. 2. (*A*) Large vegetation seen under direct visualization of ventricular lead. (*B*) Amputated leads and generator following extraction.

technique given the risk of systemic embolization across the interatrial septum. This emphasizes the importance of a complete and thorough pre-procedural workup with detailed analysis of all imaging modalities. At our center, a CT lead extraction protocol is performed in every patient and is an integral part of procedural planning. In fact, the use of electrocardiogram-gated multidetector CT has shown in the literature to often alter the approach to lead extraction and can often predict difficult cases.[12] For our patient, TTE and TEE were also crucial given the presence of endocarditis and concern for valvular pathologic condition. Another consideration regarding preoperative management and planning for our patient was thrombocytopenia. It has been reported that a low platelet count may carry a 1.7-fold increased risk of major complication during device extraction.[13] Early involvement of hematology was therefore crucial in ensuring safety of our patient in the perioperative period.

Proper evaluation of patients in the preoperative setting will undoubtedly identify a group of patients that will benefit from an open chest approach lead extraction during a percutaneous approach. These factors include patients with concomitant valvular endocarditis and pathologic condition, patients with very high risk factors for vascular perforation during a percutaneous approach, presence of a PFO, which may increase the risk of perioperative stroke, patients with considerable pulmonary embolic burden or risk for hemodynamically catastrophic emboli during an attempted percutaneous approach, and patients with concern for chronic embolic disease from indwelling transvenous leads or catheters leading to chronic thromboembolic pulmonary hypertension (CTEPH).[6,14]

SUMMARY

As the rate of CIED implantations and related infections continues to increase, percutaneous device extraction remains the preferred removal technique to reduce mortality and morbidity associated with open chest approach surgery. However, a comprehensive preprocedural workup including advanced imaging techniques may reveal the inevitable need for open chest approach extraction. Our patient presenting with CIED infection, bacteremia, large lead vegetation, and a PFO benefited from the expertise of multiple subspecialists including cardiac electrophysiology, cardiothoracic surgery, hematology, and infectious diseases at an expert, high-volume extraction center to safely undergo open chest approach lead extraction and implantation of an epicardial pacing system.

DISCLOSURE

There are no financial conflicts of interest to disclose.

SUPPLEMENTARY DATA

Supplementary data related to this article can be found online at https://doi.org/10.1016/j.ccep.2023.10.014.

REFERENCES

1. Akinyele B, Marine JE, Love C, et al. Unregulated online sales of cardiac implantable electronic devices in the United States: a six-month assessment. Heart Rhythm O2 2020;1(4):235–8.
2. Han HC, Hawkins NM, Pearman CM, et al. Epidemiology of cardiac implantable electronic device infections: incidence and risk factors. Europace 2021;23(23 Suppl 4):iv3–10.
3. Le KY, Sohail MR, Friedman PA, et al. Impact of timing of device removal on mortality in patients with cardiovascular implantable electronic device infections. Heart Rhythm 2011;8(11):1678–85.
4. Kusumoto FM, Schoenfeld MH, Wilkoff BL, et al. 2017 HRS expert consensus statement on cardiovascular implantable electronic device lead management and extraction. Heart Rhythm 2017;14(12):e503–51 [published correction appears in Heart Rhythm. 2021 Oct;18(10):1814].
5. Boarescu PM, Rosian AN, Rosian SH. Transvenous lead extraction procedure inications, methods, and complications. Biomedicines 2022;10(11):2780.
6. Wilkoff BL, Love CJ, Byrd CL, et al. Transvenous lead extraction: heart Rhythm Society expert consensus on facilities, training, indications, and patient management: this document was endorsed by the American Heart Association (AHA). Heart Rhythm 2009;6(7):1085–104.
7. Nishii N, Miyoshi A, Morimoto Y, et al. Percutaneous lead extraction for patients with large vegetations using an unusual technique. HeartRhythm Case Rep 2018;5(1):40–3.
8. Patel N, Azemi T, Zaeem F, et al. Vacuum assisted vegetation extraction for the management of large lead vegetations. J Card Surg 2013;28(3):321–4.
9. Basman C, Rashid U, Parmar YJ, et al. The role of percutaneous vacuum-assisted thrombectomy for intracardiac and intravascular pathology. J Card Surg 2018;33(10):666–72.
10. Edla S, Boshara A, Neupane S, et al. Internal jugular venous approach to percutaneous vacuum-assisted debulking of large lead vegetations prior to lead extraction. JACC Clin Electrophysiol 2018;4(1):147–8.

11. Godara H, Jia KQ, Augostini RS, et al. Feasibility of concomitant vacuum-assisted removal of lead-related vegetations and cardiac implantable electronic device extraction. J Cardiovasc Electrophysiol 2018;29(10):1460–6.
12. Lewis RK, Pokorney SD, Greenfield RA, et al. Pre-procedural ECG-gated computed tomography for prevention of complications during lead extraction. Pacing Clin Electrophysiol 2014;37(10):1297–305.
13. Brunner MP, Cronin EM, Jacob J, et al. Transvenous extraction of implantable cardioverter-defibrillator leads under advisory–a comparison of Riata, Sprint Fidelis, and non-recalled implantable cardioverter-defibrillator leads. Heart Rhythm 2013;10(10):1444–50.
14. Nayak R, Fernandes TM, Auger WR, et al. Contribution of cardiac implantable electronic devices to thrombus formation in patients with chronic thromboembolic pulmonary hypertension. JACC Clin Electrophysiol 2018;4(11):1431–6.

Micra Extraction Out To 4.5 Years

Kirollos Gabrah, DO[a,1], Arun Umesh Mahtani, MD, MS[a,b], Devi G. Nair, MD, FACC, FHRS[a,c,*]

KEYWORDS

- Leadless pacemaker • Micra transcatheter pacing system • Extraction • Retrieval

KEY POINTS

- Leadless pacemaker systems (LPs) were developed as an alternative to traditional transvenous permanent pacemakers (TV-PPM) to mitigate procedural and device-related complications.
- Two LPs are Food and Drug Administration (FDA) approved and being used commercially: Micra (Medtronic, Minneapolis, MN, USA) and Aveir (Abbott Medical, Sylmar, CA, USA).
- LPs have demonstrated low rates of complications with stable pacing performance.
- Certain clinical indications require the need for LPs to be retrieved.
- We highlight retrieval techniques of the Micra LPs and challenges encountered.

INTRODUCTION/HISTORY/BACKGROUND

The first pacemaker was implanted in the United States in June of 1960,[1] and today, it is estimated that more than 3 million people have an implantable pacemaker in the United States alone.[2] Since the 1960s, significant advancements have been made in the technology, size, weight, battery life, and leads of the pacemaker systems. The goal has always been to have the smallest device that is easy to implant with the longest battery life and the lowest possible risk of infection. In April 2016, the Food and Drug Administration (FDA) approved the Micra transcatheter pacing system, a leadless pacemaker system (LPs), approximately the size of an AAA battery, which is implanted in the right ventricle (**Fig. 1**).

NATURE OF THE PROBLEM/DIAGNOSIS

LPs started to be in favor especially with recent trials showing 38% lower rates of reinterventions and 31% lower rates of chronic complications.[3] They also became in favor for patients that had prior issues during the placement of the traditional transvenous permanent pacemaker (TV-PPM).[4] Retrieval of LPs becomes a consideration when the pacemaker's battery life is depleted, in cases of device malfunction, dislodgement, upgrades, or infection where multiple retrieval techniques and tools come in handy.

ANATOMY

The Micra LPs consists of a retrieval feature located at the proximal end, 4 nitinol tines at the distal end, an anode, and a cathode (**Fig. 2**). The Micra LPs is implanted into the right ventricular septum and is tethered to the right ventricle using the 4 nitinol tines.

PREOPERATIVE PLANNING

Both Micra VR and Micra AV devices were designed to provide both implanters and patients with options regarding retrieval. They can potentially be left in place and the device can be programmed off and a new Micra can be implanted or a traditional system can be implanted if needed.

[a] Arrhythmia Research Group, Jonesboro, AR, USA; [b] Department of Internal Medicine, 355 Bard Avenue, Staten Island, NY 10310, USA; [c] Department of Electrophysiology, St. Bernards Medical Center, Jonesboro, AR, USA
[1] Present address. 201 East Oak Avenue, Jonesboro, AR 72401, USA.
* Corresponding author. 201 East Oak Avenue, Jonesboro, AR 72401, USA.
E-mail address: drdevignair@gmail.com
Twitter: @drdevignair (D.G.N.)

Card Electrophysiol Clin 16 (2024) 149–155
https://doi.org/10.1016/j.ccep.2023.10.015
1877-9182/24/© 2023 Elsevier Inc. All rights reserved.

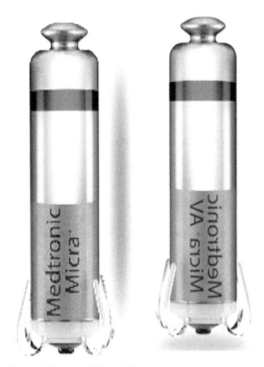

Fig. 1. Micra and Micra AV.

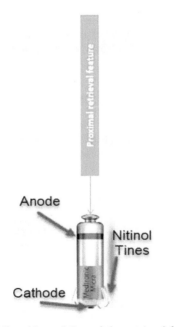

Fig. 2. Micra LP consisting of the retrieval feature, 4 nitinol tines, an anode, and a cathode.

If the device needs to be removed then the proximal retrieval feature enables acute retrieval.

PREPARATION AND PATIENT POSITIONING

The patient is placed in a supine position. The right groin is sterilized using chlorhexidine and/or betadine. Sedation is administered to the patient. The right femoral vein is visualized using vascular ultrasonography to obtain sheath access.

PROCEDURAL APPROACH

Once patient preparation is complete, 2 approaches have currently been described for acute retrieval (<6 weeks of implantation) of the Micra LPs.[5]

The first approach uses the Micra introducer and delivery system with a compatible snare.

1. Through the first right-sided femoral venous access, the Micra introducer sheath is inserted. This is a 27Fr nonsteerable sheath with hydrophilic coating allowing for smooth vessel entry.
2. Through the Micra introducer sheath, the Micra delivery system is introduced. This is a 23Fr catheter with dual purpose of implantation as well as retrieval of the Micra LPs. It is a deflectable catheter of up to 120° deflection consisting of a handle and a distal end (**Fig. 3**). The handle consists of a control system to steer the catheter. The distal end consists of an inner and outer shaft, a device cup, and a recapture cone.
3. A single or tri-loop snare is inserted through the Micra delivery system. Various sizes ranging from 7 to 10 mm may be used.
4. The recapture cone is placed close to the proximal retrieval feature of the Micra, and the snare is deployed (**Fig. 4**). Traction from the snare and countertraction from the recapture cone leads to stretching of the nitinol tines and dislodgement of the system from the myocardium. The delivery catheter, Micra LPs, and introducer sheath are all withdrawn from the patient.

The second approach uses a Micra introducer system with a steerable introducer sheath and a gooseneck snare for better coaxial positioning to engage the proximal retrieval feature (**Fig. 5**).

1. After femoral venous access, the Micra introducer sheath is inserted.
2. Next a shorter sheath is introduced into the introducer sheath (12–16Fr) to allow for hemostasis across the valve on the Micra sheath.
3. A steerable sheath such as an Agilis NXT (Abbott Medical, Sylmar, CA, USA) is advanced

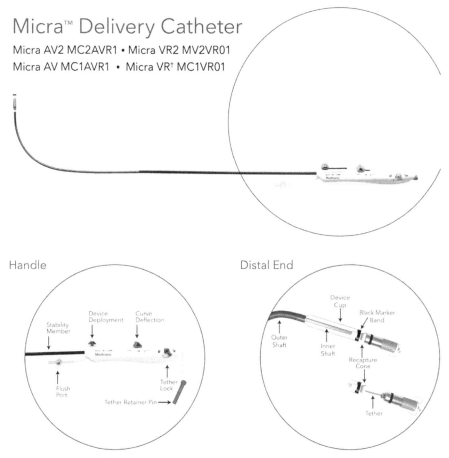

Micra™ Delivery Catheter

Micra AV2 MC2AVR1 • Micra VR2 MV2VR01
Micra AV MC1AVR1 • Micra VR† MC1VR01

Handle

Stability Member
Device Deployment
Curve Deflection
Flush Port
Tether Retainer Pin
Tether Lock

Distal End

Device Cup
Black Marker Band
Outer Shaft
Inner Shaft
Recapture Cone
Tether

Fig. 3. Micra delivery catheter showing the handle and distal end. (Images used with permission from Medtronic, plc © 2023.)

into the right atrium and right ventricle over a wire.

4. Through the Agilis, a gooseneck snare (Minimum 10–20 mm loop) or a single/tri-loop snare can be advanced to the proximal retrieval feature of the Micra. Once the proximal retrieval feature is engaged, traction can be allowed to facilitate the release of the tines and dislodgement of the pacing capsule from the myocardium.

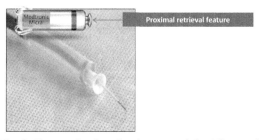
Proximal retrieval feature

Fig. 4. The proximal retrieval system of the Micra and recapture cone.

5. The Micra LPs along with the sheaths are all withdrawn from the patient.

Certain challenges can be encountered during the retrieval process such as the following:

1. Off axis plane of the Micra LPs
2. Complete dislodgement of the Micra LPs
3. Chordae tendinae or moderator band limiting access to the proximal retrieval feature
4. Encapsulation
1. Coaxial orientation needs to be ensured during the retrieval process to successfully guide the Micra LPs into the sheaths. In case of an off-axis plane, the snare can be wrapped around the body of the Micra LPs instead of the proximal retrieval feature to facilitate coaxial orientation. Moreover, 2 snares can be used via a separate venous access to successfully orient, capture, and guide the Micra LPs into the sheaths (**Fig. 6**).[6]
2. In cases of complete dislodgement of the Micra LPs, several techniques can be used to retrieve

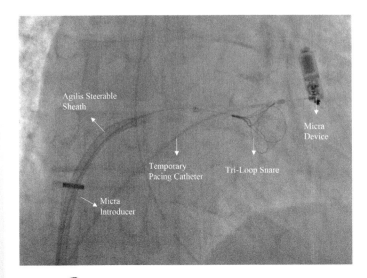

Fig. 5. Micra retrieval using agilis.

Agilis Steerable
Sheath

Micra
Device

Temporary
Pacing Catheter

Tri-Loop Snare

Micra
Introducer

the device. In addition to the single-loop, tri-loop, and double snare techniques, other retrievers such as the INARI Flowtriever (Inari Medical, Irvine, CA, USA; **Fig. 7**) and the ONO retrieval device (ONOCOR LLC, Philadelphia, PA, USA) can also be used (**Fig. 8**).[7–9]

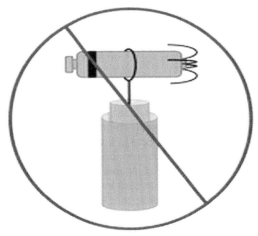

Fig. 6. Off axis Micra.

- The INARI Flowtriever is a 24Fr sheath, which is used to perform aspiration thrombectomy of pulmonary emboli and can be used to retrieve dislodged Micra LPs into the pulmonary artery. An Amplatz super stiff guidewire (Boston Scientific, Marlborough, MA, USA) can be used to maintain access in the pulmonary vasculature. Two 20 mm gooseneck snares (one through the T24 Flowtriever system) should be used to

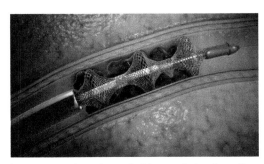

Fig. 7. INARI Flowtriever. (With permission from Flow-Triever® System, Inari Medical.)

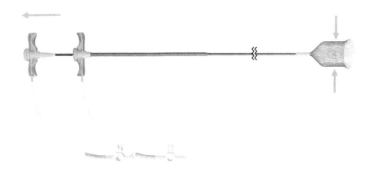

Fig. 8. ONO retrieval device. (With permission from The ONO device, ONOCOR Vascular.)

secure the device and direct it into the main pulmonary artery through the Flowtriever system.[8]

- The ONO retrieval device is a 12Fr device fused with a 7Fr catheter containing a series nitinol loops to form a basket-like trap that received FDA approval in 2022. McNamara and colleagues describes a case of a 52-year-old woman who had a Micra LPs migrate to the right posterolateral trunk of the pulmonary venous system. Because of inadequate luminal space and healing of the device, snaring could not be performed and instead a 10 × 20 mm Armada (Abbott, Sylmar, CA, USA) balloon was inflated distal to the device and retracted, which led to the device dislodging into the proximal right pulmonary artery. The distal flange was snared, and the Micra LP was captured by the ONO

retrieval device allowing for easy removal from the patient's body.[7]

3. In case of chordae tendinae or moderator band limiting access to the proximal retrieval feature, intracardiac echocardiography (ICE) through a separate venous access can be used to directly visualize the retrieval feature facilitating successful extraction of the Micra LPs.[10,11]

- Moreover, in several cases, the Aveir retrieval catheter system (Abbott Medical, Sylmar, CA, USA) has been used to retrieve the Micra pacing capsule. The Aveir retrieval system has a steerable, deflectable, delivery catheter with an integrated guiding catheter that houses a tri-loop snare, which allows us to dock the Micra retrieval feature. There is a protective sleeve that can fully cover the Micra system and prevent any chordae from getting in the way. This also reduces the risk of injury to other cardiovascular structures from the snare during retraction (**Fig. 9**). This technique uses a 27Fr introducer into the femoral vein. The triple loop snare within the Aveir retrieval system is used for engaging the proximal retrieval feature on the Micra. The protective sleeve is advanced over the docked device and countertraction is applied until the device disengages from the myocardium and is pulled back into the sheath to ensure safe retrieval.[12–14]

4. Finally, in cases where the device has been encapsulated, a Bioptome or Raptor (Diagmed Healthcare, North Yorkshire, England) toothed forceps catheter can be used to expose the proximal retrieval feature.

5. The decision to retrieve the device needs to be considered based on risks/benefits and indications. Retrieval can result in cardiac injury including myocardial avulsion.[5] In such scenarios, leaving the device in situ and turning off the device to OOO/OFF mode may be a suitable and safe option.[5,15,16]

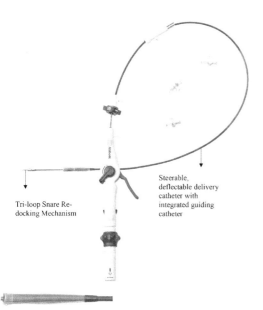

Tri-loop Snare Re-docking Mechanism

Steerable, deflectable delivery catheter with integrated guiding catheter

Fig. 9. Aveir retrieval catheter system and the protective sleeve.

RECOVERY AND REHABILITATION

Retrieval of the Micra LPs is a percutaneous procedure through the femoral veins. Bleeding at access sites is either controlled by applying pressure or closed with suture-mediated systems. The patient can be discharged home the same day or may stay in the hospital overnight for observation.

OUTCOMES

More than 200,000 LPs have been implanted worldwide, and implantation rates will only continue to increase with the development of newer versions to accommodate more pacing indications. Several studies have reported a relatively safe outcome of this procedure irrespective of the duration of the implantation.[17,18] Acute retrievals were attributed to increasing thresholds and dislodgement, whereas delayed retrievals were related to increased capture threshold, device upgrade, and infection.[5,17]

SUMMARY

This review highlights the different procedural steps and techniques for the retrieval of the Micra LPs. Different procedural challenges and ways to counter them have also been mentioned.

CLINICS CARE POINTS

1. Consider risk/benefits and indication for retrieval.
2. Consider the lifetime of the patient.
3. Commonly used option: Single/Tri-loop snare or Gooseneck snare with deflectable sheath within Micra introducer sheath.
4. Can use nontraditional strategies in case of dislodged devices.
   - Double snare
   - Bioptome/raptor
   - Aveir retrieval catheter
   - ICE guidance to direct toward proximal retrieval feature.
   - INARI thrombectomy aspiration catheter or ONO basket retrieval system.

FUNDING

There were no associated grants, contracts, or other forms of financial support.

DISCLOSURE

Kirollos Gabrah, DO: The author has nothing to disclose. Arun Umesh Mahtani, MD, MS: The author has nothing to disclose. Devi Nair, MD: The author has received grants, research support, consulting fees, or honoraria from Boston Scientific Corp, Medtronic Inc, Abbott Medical, Biosense Webster, Adagio, and Affera.

REFERENCES

1. Beck H, Boden WE, Patibandla S, et al. 50th Anniversary of the first successful permanent pacemaker implantation in the United States: historical review and future directions. Am J Cardiol 2010;106(6): 810–8.
2. Benjamin MM, Sorkness CA. Practical and ethical considerations in the management of pacemaker and implantable cardiac defibrillator devices in terminally ill patients. Proc (Bayl Univ Med Cent) 2017;30(2):157–60.
3. El-Chami MF, Bockstedt L, Longacre C, et al. Leadless vs. transvenous single-chamber ventricular pacing in the Micra CED study: 2-year follow-up. Eur Heart J 2022;43(12):1207–15.
4. Seriwala HM, Khan MS, Munir MB, et al. Leadless pacemakers: a new era in cardiac pacing. J Cardiol 2016;67(1):1–5.
5. Afzal MR, Daoud EG, Cunnane R, et al. Techniques for successful early retrieval of the Micra transcatheter pacing system: a worldwide experience. Heart Rhythm 2018;15(6):841–6.
6. Goyal R, Markowitz SM, Ip JE. Double-snare technique for capturing a wandering leadless pacemaker. JACC (J Am Coll Cardiol): Clinical Electrophysiology 2019;5(7):872–3.
7. McNamara GP, Haber ZM, Lee EW, et al. Successful removal of a leadless pacemaker from the pulmonary artery via a novel basket retrieval system. HeartRhythm Case Reports 2023;9(4):215–8.
8. Gupta S, Cho K, Papagiannis J, et al. A novel technique for extraction of a leadless pacemaker that embolized to the pulmonary artery in a young patient: a case report. HeartRhythm Case Reports 2020;6(10):724–8.
9. Romeo E, D'Alto M, Cappelli M, et al. Retrieval of a leadless transcatheter pacemaker from the right pulmonary artery: a case report. Pacing Clin Electrophysiol 2021;44(5):952–4.
10. Kiani S, Merchant FM, El-Chami MF. Extraction of a 4-year-old leadless pacemaker with a tine-based fixation. HeartRhythm Case Reports 2019;5(8): 424–5.
11. Ellison K, Hesselson A, Ayoub K, et al. Retrieval of an infected leadless pacemaker. HeartRhythm Case Reports 2020;6(11):863–6.

12. Callahan IVTD, Wilkoff BL. Extraction of a 5-year-old leadless pacemaker using a competing manufacturer's removal tool. HeartRhythm Case Reports 2023;9(7):441–4.

13. Jain V, Shah AD, Lloyd MS. Need for a universal retrieval tool with countertraction for the removal of leadless pacemakers regardless of the manufacturer. Heart Rhythm 2023;20(7):1068–9.

14. Lee B, Doty B, Brider J, et al. PO-04-008 NOVEL APPROACH TO LEADLESS MEDTRONIC MICRATM PACEMAKER EXTRACTION WITH ABBOTT AVEIRTMVR VENTRICULAR RETRIEVAL CATHETER SYSTEM. Heart Rhythm 2023;20(5):S582–3. https://doi.org/10.1016/j.hrthm.2023.03.1233.

15. Grubman E, Ritter P, Ellis CR, et al. To retrieve, or not to retrieve: system revisions with the Micra transcatheter pacemaker. Heart Rhythm 2017; 14(12):1801–6.

16. Duray GZ, Ritter P, El-Chami M, et al. Long-term performance of a transcatheter pacing system: 12-month results from the Micra Transcatheter Pacing Study. Heart Rhythm 2017;14(5):702–9.

17. Dar T, Akella K, Murtaza G, et al. Comparison of the safety and efficacy of Nanostim and Micra transcatheter leadless pacemaker (LP) extractions: a multicenter experience. J Intervent Card Electrophysiol 2020;57:133–40.

18. Karim S, Abdelmessih M, Marieb M, et al. Extraction of a Micra transcatheter pacing system: first-in-human experience. HeartRhythm Case Reports 2016;2(1):60–2.

Severe Tricuspid Regurgitation in a Patient with a Transvenous Dual-chamber Pacemaker
Considerations for Diagnosis and Management

Sami H. Ibrahim, MD, Pamela K. Mason, MD*

KEYWORDS

- Tricuspid regurgitation • Lead extraction • Leadless pacing
- Cardiac implantable electronic devices

KEY POINTS

- Transvenous pacemaker and defibrillator leads can contribute to tricuspid regurgitation.
- Extraction of transvenous leads alone is usually not enough to resolve the tricuspid regurgitation due to right ventricular remodeling and leaflet adhesions.
- There are risks to jailing transvenous leads during tricuspid valve procedures.
- There are alternative pacing and defibrillation methods to traditional transvenous leads that can help with management for patients with severe tricuspid regurgitation.

CASE PRESENTATION

Mr W is a 78 year-old man with past medical history of atrial fibrillation, hypothyroidism, hypertension, prior tobacco abuse, sinus node dysfunction (SND), and complete heart block (CHB) who had a dual-chamber pacemaker placed in 2015 (Medtronic, pacing leads-model 5076). Before pacer placement, cardiac MRI showed normal left ventricular (LV) function, moderate reduction in right ventricular (RV) function, and mild tricuspid regurgitation (TR). In January 2023, he was admitted for decompensated heart failure (HF). Before this, he had several admissions for acute decompensated HF with preserved ejection fraction (EF); however, he was now found to have an EF of 45% to 50%, systolic and diastolic flattening of the ventricular septum consistent with RV pressure and volume overload, and severe TR with a dilated tricuspid

valve (TV) annulus (**Fig. 1**). The cause of his worsened TR was thought to be a combination of functional due to RV dysfunction and tricuspid annulus dilation and impingement from the RV pacing lead. He received diuretic therapy and was discharged.

He was seen by a cardiothoracic surgeon the following week to discuss further management options for his severe TR. With his otherwise stable comorbidities, he was planned for an open TV replacement. The electrophysiology service was asked for recommendations for preoperative management of his device because he remained pacemaker dependent with severe SND and CHB. A multidisciplinary plan was made to perform extraction of the RV lead, convert the dual-chamber transvenous pacing system to a right atrial (RA) pacing system, and place a leadless pacemaker (Medtronic Micra AV, Minneapolis, MN). Thus, the patient would pace the RA via the transvenous

University of Virginia, Box 800158, Charlottesville, VA 22908, USA
* Corresponding author.
E-mail address: PKM5F@uvahealth.org

Card Electrophysiol Clin 16 (2024) 157–161
https://doi.org/10.1016/j.ccep.2023.10.016
1877-9182/24/© 2023 Elsevier Inc. All rights reserved.

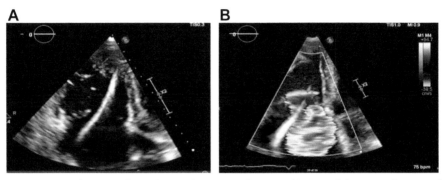

Fig. 1. Preoperative transthoracic echocardiography images showing dilation of the RV and TV annulus (*A*) and severe TR (*B*).

system and the leadless device would track the atrium to maintain atrio-ventricular (AV) synchrony. After these procedures, the TV replacement would be performed surgically.

Lead extraction was performed in early February 2023 with the RV pacing lead extracted, the RA lead left in place, and the generator changed to a single-chamber generator (Medtronic Azure XT SR, Minneapolis, MN) programmed to AAIR mode. A leadless pacemaker (Medtronic Micra AV, Minneapolis, MN) was subsequently placed without any procedural complications (**Fig. 2**). A device interrogation of the leadless pacemaker the following day showed elevated thresholds but with appropriate pacing and tracking of the atria. The postextraction echocardiogram also showed persistent malcoaptation of the TV leaflets with minimal improvement in TR after lead extraction (**Fig. 3**). He was discharged in good condition with the TV replacement scheduled at the end of the month.

At the end of February, cardiothoracic surgery successfully placed a 33-mm Abbott Epic Plus porcine TV (Santa Clara, CA) with no significant residual leak. Due to the high threshold on the leadless pacemaker, it was elected to place an epicardial LV lead for pacing. During the procedure, the single-chamber generator was exchanged with a dual-chamber system (Medtronic Azure XT DR, Minneapolis, MN), and an epicardial ventricular lead was sutured onto the LV apex, tunneled into the pacemaker pocket, and connected to the new generator along with the chronic RA lead. The leadless pacemaker was abandoned. His postop course was complicated by RV failure requiring aggressive diuresis, milrinone, and inhaled nitric oxide but both agents were soon weaned off and his clinical status improved until he was stable for discharge. His left ventricular ejection fraction (LVEF) improved to 50% to 55% after surgery.

Six months after this, the patient presented to the emergency department with palpitations and syncope. He was found to be in ventricular tachycardia, defibrillation was emergently performed, and the patient was recommended for a secondary prevention implantable cardioverter-defibrillator (ICD) after evaluation revealed no reversible causes. The patient was concerned about having his TV crossed again with another, even larger lead. He failed screening for a subcutaneous ICD, and there was additional concern about oversensing with this device due to his epicardial pacing lead. After a discussion, a request was made for compassionate use of the investigational Medtronic novel ICD lead, which is lumenless and 4.7 French in size, nearly half the diameter of most commercially available ICD leads.[1]

CONTRIBUTION OF TRANSVENOUS RIGHT VENTRICULAR LEADS TO TRICUSPID REGURGITATION

The cause for new or worsening TR may be ambiguous in patients with cardiac implantable electronic device (CIEDs).[2,3] TR in non-CIED patients is usually functional and worsens as the RV becomes more dilated due to volume overload or chronically elevated pulmonary pressures. In patients with CIEDs, lead-induced TR can occur acutely after implantation from direct trauma-causing leaflet perforation, avulsion, or damage to the subvalvular apparatus. In addition, lead impingement of one of the tricuspid leaflets can result in malcoaptation. Those who are more at risk include patients with larger diameter ICD leads, multiple RV leads in place, and those with baseline RV dysfunction or a dilated annulus. With long-term RV pacing, there may also be changes in the RV structure over time, contributing to the progression of functional TR with annular

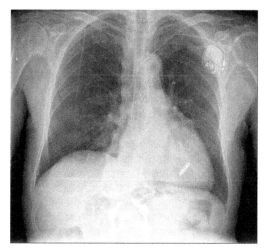

Fig. 2. Chest radiograph after RV lead extraction and leadless pacemaker placement.

dilation and leaflet tethering, eventually reaching a severity and mechanism that is independent of the lead itself. Although the TR usually begins as a trace-to-mild severity, this can later worsen significantly as the RV continues to dilate. A 2018 prospective study demonstrated a 5% increase in the prevalence of moderate-to-severe TR 1 year after lead implantation.[4] The severity of TR is often diagnosed with either transthoracic echocardiogram or transesophageal echocardiogram; however, in those with transvenous leads, the degree of TR may be underestimated if the TR is an eccentric wall-hugging jet with loss of Doppler color flow (Coanda effect) or if there is imaging artifact from the lead itself.[2] This can ultimately lead to a delay in diagnosis. Acute management of worsening TR initially involves volume optimization with diuresis

but eventually valve replacement and further lead management will need to be considered.

BENEFITS OF LEAD EXTRACTION FOR TRICUSPID REGURGITATION

Lead extraction is sometimes considered in the setting of worsening HF and significant TR that is thought to be directly related to the transvenous RV lead.[5] There are no large studies to guide recommendations with regards to lead extraction in these circumstances and published recommendations are mostly based on expert opinion.[3] The outcomes of lead extraction and the degree of improvement of the TR are variable and likely dependent on the mechanism of the TR, the degree of RV remodeling, and the age of the leads. Newer implants associated with acute lead impingement are more likely to have improvement after extraction as RV remodeling and adhesions of the TV apparatus would not yet have occurred. If this is the case, lead extraction may be feasible alone without needing surgical interventions. With older leads, extraction is less likely to lead to acute improvement in the TR. For long-standing TR with associated annular dilation and valve impingement, leaflet coaptation likely will not be possible even after removing or repositioning the lead. There is also a chance that the lead extraction itself may cause more valvular damage and worsen the TR, and there should be a tricuspid valve intervention strategy in place at the time of lead extraction.[6] Lead removal and revision can also be done surgically at the time of valve repair. The timing becomes more complicated if the patient is pacemaker dependent or has an ICD lead in place. Overall, when considering lead extraction to assist in the management of TR, it is crucial to

A 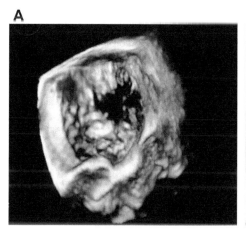 **B**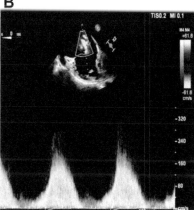

Fig. 3. Transthoracic echocardiography after RV lead extraction. Persistent malcoaptation of the valve leaflets is still present by three-dimensional images (*A*) and continuous wave Doppler jet demonstrates continued severe TR (*B*).

factor in the chronicity of the TR, the degree of RV enlargement and TV annular dilation, the degree of RV dysfunction, and if significant TV leaflet damage is present. Consideration also needs to be made as to the patient's candidacy for valve interventions as well as their device needs. Finally, even if extraction is not likely to improve TR, it can be indicated before a planned TV procedure to prevent jailing of leads.

JAILING TRANSVENOUS LEADS DURING TRICUSPID VALVE PROCEDURES

A jailed lead is a transvenous lead that is entrapped against the tricuspid annulus or an older surgical valve by the hardware of a tricuspid replacement or repair.[7] Management of transvenous pacing leads around the time of TV interventions, including both open surgical and transcatheter repair or replacement, has been an area of controversy. Although some case series have described minimal damage and normal function of jailed leads at follow-up, there are not extensive data to support this practice.[8] There are also some data suggesting a risk of significant damage and lead malfunction.[9,10] Furthermore, extraction of those damaged leads after the TV replacement can become extremely difficult and often ultimately require surgical removal.[11] It becomes more complicated when these patients are pacemaker dependent or have an ICD lead that could result in inappropriate shocks if there is a fracture. In these certain patient populations, it has been proposed to perform the lead extraction beforehand to avoid jailing, replace the valve, and then determine the most appropriate strategy and timing for new pacing or ICD lead placement for each patient. If the goal is to avoid crossing a surgically replaced TV, whether it be by using a leadless pacemaker beforehand (as in our patient), epicardial pacing lead placement, subcutaneous ICD lead placement, or the coronary sinus for either pacing or ICD leads. Ultimately, these patients benefit greatly from a detailed preprocedure planning strategy between the structural cardiologist or cardiothoracic surgeon and the electrophysiologist before the valve replacement.[3]

COMPLEX DEVICE SYSTEMS IN THE SETTING OF RECENT TRICUSPID VALVE REPLACEMENTS

Alternative approaches to transvenous leads have been discussed in the literature when confronted with a newly placed bioprosthetic TV. Although nonmechanical valves can be crossed, it is often desired to avoid this, especially if a lead was thought to be the original cause of TR. To provide pacing, the primary options to provide RV pacing involve a leadless pacing system, a pacing lead placed within the coronary sinus, or epicardial pacing leads placed during surgery. To provide defibrillation, options include a subcutaneous ICD or possibly a defibrillation coil into the coronary sinus. In patients who are pacemaker dependent and also have an indication for an ICD, a combination of options may need to be considered. If there are epicardial pacing wires in place, it might be difficult to successfully place a subcutaneous ICD, and a coil in the coronary sinus could be used instead. A leadless pacemaker can be paired with a subcutaneous ICD, although there are important programming considerations when pairing different devices.[12] With newer generation leads being manufactured, more options will likely develop in the future. For this patient, the team was able to provide AV synchronous pacing without crossing the TV through combinations of transvenous atrial pacing, leadless pacing, and ultimately, epicardial RV pacing. After he experienced sustained ventricular tachycardia, his options to avoid crossing the new valve were limited and compassionate use of a novel, small diameter, ICD lead was requested.[1]

SUMMARY

Patients with severe TR, HF, and transvenous RV leads are a heterogenous group, and one management strategy will not work for every patient. Even if the lead is mechanically contributing to the TR, removal of chronic leads often does not improve the TR due to annular dilation and adhesions of the valvular apparatus. If planning for extraction, careful consideration must be given as to the specific mechanisms of the TR, the age and type of the RV lead, procedural risks, pacing and defibrillator needs, as well as patient preferences. A multidisciplinary approach involving cardiac surgery, electrophysiology, imaging, and HF services is ideal when valve intervention is planned. With modern and safer extraction procedures, extraction to avoid jailing leads is ideal when possible. Newer leadless and subcutaneous device options give patients more options to avoid crossing the TV.

CLINICS CARE POINTS

- Care should be taken when placing right ventriuclar transvenous leads to avoid tricuspid valve inpindgment.

- Patients with CIEDs and severe tricuspid regurgitation require a multi-displinary apporach to manage the valve, device needs, and heart failure.
- Jailing of transvenous right ventriular pacing leads during tricuspid valve interventions should be avoided.
- CIED patients with severe tricuspid regurgiation should be managed at centers with high volume extraction and structural heart experience.

DISCLOSURE

Dr Mason provides consulting services to and receives honoaria from Medtronic and Boston Scientific; Dr Ibrahim has no disclosures.

ACKNOWLEDGMENT

There are no acknowedgments.

REFERENCES

1. Crossley GH, Sanders P, De Filippo P, et al. Rationale and design of the lead evaluation for defibrillation and reliability study: safety and efficacy of a novel ICD lead design. J Cardiovasc Electrophysiol 2023;34(2):257–67. Epub 2023 Jan 8. Erratum in: J Cardiovasc Electrophysiol. 2023 Sep;34(9): 2011.

2. Chang JD, Manning WJ, Ebrille E, et al. Tricuspid valve dysfunction following pacemaker or cardioverter-defibrillator implantation. J Am Coll Cardiol 2017; 69(18):2331–41.

3. Vij A, Kavinsky CJ. The clinical impact of device lead-associated tricuspid regurgitation: need for a multidisciplinary approach. Circulation 2022; 145(4):239–41.

4. Van De Heyning CM, Elbarasi E, Masiero S, et al. Prospective study of tricuspid regurgitation associated with permanent leads after cardiac rhythm device implantation. Can J Cardiol 2019;35(4):389–95.

5. Khor L, Madan K, Lee CH, et al. Pacing lead extraction in the management of tricuspid regurgitation: a case report. Eur Heart J Case Rep 2022;6(7): ytac170.

6. Polewczyk A, Jacheć W, Nowosielecka D, et al. Tricuspid valve damage related to transvenous lead extraction. Int J Environ Res Public Health 2022;19(19):12279.

7. Schaller RD, Giri J, Epstein AE. Entrapped leads after transcatheter tricuspid valve replacement. JACC Cardiovasc Interv 2021;14(6):715–6.

8. Anderson JH, McElhinney DB, Aboulhosn J, et al. Management and outcomes of transvenous pacing leads in patients undergoing transcatheter tricuspid valve replacement. JACC Cardiovasc Interv 2020; 13(17):2012–20.

9. O'Riordan, M. (2023, June 5). Serious risks with 'jailing' pacemaker, ICD Leads during TTVR. TCTMD. Retrieved September 10, 2023. Available at: https://tctmd.com/news/serious-risks-jailing-pacemaker-icd-leads-during-TTVR.

10. Ibrahim R, Bhatia N, Merchant FM, et al. Managing transvenous right ventricular leads in the era of transcatheter tricuspid valve interventions. HeartRhythm Case Rep 2022;8(10):692–4.

11. Paz Rios LH, Alsaad AA, Guerrero M, et al. Tricuspid valve-in-valve jailing right ventricular lead is not free of risk. Catheter Cardiovasc Interv 2020;96(7): E758–60.

12. Porterfield C, DiMarco JP, Mason PK. Effectiveness of implantation of a subcutaneous implantable cardioverter-defibrillator in a patient with complete heart block and a pacemaker. Am J Cardiol 2015; 115(2):276–8.

Accidental Conduction System Pacing in Patient with Displaced Cardiac Resynchronization Therapy Leads

Vidish Pandya, MD[a], Andrew Krumerman, MD[b],*

KEYWORDS

- Conduction system pacing • Cardiac resynchronization therapy • Right bundle branch block
- Interrogation • Remote monitoring

KEY POINTS

- Cardiac resynchronization therapy (CRT) has historically been the standard of care for ventricular dyssynchrony, but recent evidence suggests CSP, specifically His bundle pacing and left bundle branch area pacing, could offer similar benefits, especially when CRT lead placement proves challenging.
- A shift toward remote monitoring of cardiac implantable electronic devices (CIEDs) with alert based follow-up will help ease burden on electrophysiology clinics.
- CIED troubleshooting requires an appropriate clinical setting and proper tools in order to adequately elucidate and resolve problems that arise.

INTRODUCTION

Cardiac implantable electronic devices (CIEDs) have witnessed a surge in global utilization, reflecting both the expanding body of literature attesting to their benefits in various cardiovascular conditions and improved worldwide accessibility. Current data indicate that the global implantation rate exceeds 1.7 million devices annually.[1] As the indications for these devices become increasingly refined and more patients are offered these therapies, it becomes crucial to have consistent follow-up and management to ensure their optimal functionality and longevity. For years, the gold standard mandated at-minimum annual consultations in electrophysiology clinic for this. Despite advancements in remote monitoring (RM) capabilities, a notable reluctance persisted among patients to embrace this technology. However, the unprecedented circumstances of the COVID-19 pandemic necessitated a shift in this paradigm that may benefit both patients and electrophysiology (EP) clinics.

Currently, a wealth of data supports the use of implantable cardioverter-defibrillators (ICDs) in heart failure with reduced ejection fraction (HFrEF) and it remains a Class I american heart association (AHA)/american college of cardiology (ACC)/heart failure society of america (HFSA) recommendation for primary prevention of sudden cardiac death in a significant number of patients with this diagnosis.[2] Furthermore, there is compelling evidence that supports cardiac resynchronization therapy (CRT) for improving symptoms and mortality in a specific subset of patients. The objective of CRT is to restore synchronized mechanical function to the left ventricle as if native conduction was intact.

a Department of Medicine, Montefiore Medical Center, 111 Ease 210th Street, Bronx, NY 10467, USA;
b Montefiore-Einstein Center for Heart and Vascular Care, Montefiore Medical Center, 111 East 210th Street, Forman 2 Cardiology, Bronx, NY 10467, USA
* Corresponding author.
E-mail address: akrumerm@montefiore.org

Card Electrophysiol Clin 16 (2024) 163–168
https://doi.org/10.1016/j.ccep.2023.10.017
1877-9182/24/© 2023 Elsevier Inc. All rights reserved.

cardiacEP.theclinics.com

Conduction system pacing (CSP) has emerged as a promising alternative to CRT. In this article, the authors present a unique case of a patient who unintentionally received CSP, along with a review of guidelines on CRT, CSP, and best practices of device management.

CASE PRESENTATION

A 69-year-old woman with a history of nonischemic cardiomyopathy and HFrEF with an left ventricular ejection fraction (LVEF) of 35% presented to electrophysiology clinic for first time device interrogation. She had a Medtronic CRT ICD implanted 11 years prior in Puerto Rico for primary prevention and not had her device checked for several years. Despite the lack of follow-up, she was presumed to be faring well until a recent hospitalization where she was found to have systolic heart failure (HF), depressed LVEF, and severe functional mitral regurgitation.

ECG at the time of presentation to the office (**Fig. 1**) displayed an atrial-sensed, ventricular-paced rhythm with a ventricular rate of 80 beats per minute and a QRS duration of 120 millisecond.

Device interrogation showed adequate pacing thresholds, sensing, and impedance values for the atrial and right ventricular (ICD) leads. The left ventricular lead, however, achieved ventricular capture at 8 V at 0.5 millisecond and atrial capture only at lower outputs. RV only pacing demonstrated a left bundle, left axis morphology with a QRS duration of 140 millisecond. Underlying rhythm demonstrated normal sinus rhythm with

right bundle branch block (RBBB), a PR interval of 168 millisecond, and a QRS duration of 158 millisecond (**Fig. 2**).

Concerns arising from the LV lead interrogation prompted a chest X-ray (**Fig. 3**). The imaging revealed downward migration of the pulse generator sitting at the level of the left lower lung field. All leads had retracted toward the shoulder. The proximal portion of the SVC coil was adjacent to the junction of the left axillary and left subclavian veins. The atrial lead, devoid of its J curve, was in contact with the high right atrial wall, and the LV lead was situated with its tip in the proximal coronary sinus (CS). Owing to the LV lead's position and its high pacing thresholds, it was deemed ineffective and was subsequently programmed off.

Interestingly, the patient's initial ECG demonstrated a narrow QRS despite her underlying RBBB pattern. This finding suggested that the RV lead was retracted in a manner where its tip was positioned somewhere along the basilar interventricular septum near the right bundle branch. Pacing from the RV lead (in ventricular pacing mode [VVI] mode) produced a relatively narrow QRS with left bundle morphology. In dual chamber pacing mode (DDD) mode, the RV lead's capture of the right bundle combined with the intact intrinsic left bundle branch conduction further shortened the QRS duration to 126 milliseconds, and the RBBB pattern was no longer noted.

Following a detailed discussion regarding possible lead extraction/revision, the patient declined any intervention. She underwent noninvasive programmed stimulation and defibrillation

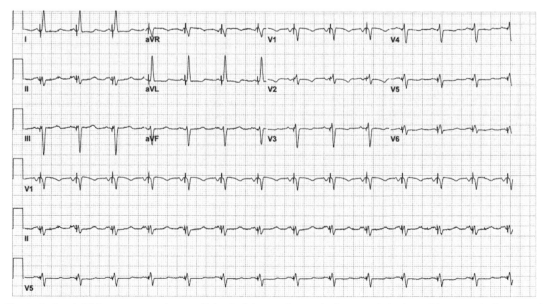

Fig. 1. Patient's ECG on presentation to clinic. Atrial-sensed, ventricular-paced rhythm with a ventricular rate of 80 beats per minute and a QRS duration of 120 millisecond.

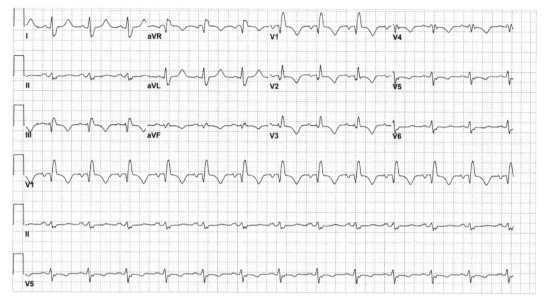

Fig. 2. ECG of patient's underlying rhythm. Normal sinus rhythm with right bundle branch block. PR interval of 168 millisecond and a QRS duration of 158 millisecond.

threshold testing. Burst pacing at 50 Hz induced ventricular fibrillation, which was promptly detected and terminated with a 25-J shock. This confirmed functionality of the RV lead to defibrillate effectively.

The device was programmed to DDD 50 to 130 beats per minute (with RV pacing only). Ventricular tachycardia (VT) monitor zone was set to 176 bpm and ventricular fibrillation (VF) zone was set at 194 bpm. Given appropriate RV pacing and adequate defibrillation threshold testing, there was no immediate need for device revision or replacement, and biannual follow-up was planned.

Over the ensuing year, the HF team closely managed the patient due to her challenges in maintaining a euvolemic state. She underwent evaluation by the structural heart team for potential mitral valve repair. However, with meticulous titration of guideline-directed medical therapy

(GDMT), her mitral regurgitation improved, leading to a decision to defer the repair. Echocardiogram demonstrated mild mitral regurgitation and an LVEF of 55%. Throughout this period, her rhythm persisted as atrial-sensed and ventricular-paced, with 99% RV pacing.

DISCUSSION
Cardiac Resynchronization Therapy Versus Conduction System Pacing

Cardiac physiologic pacing aims to maintain or restore the synchrony of ventricular contraction and can be achieved through two primary methods.

1. Cardiac resynchronization therapy: This method typically uses biventricular (BiV) pacing and involves the use of a CS branch lead or an epicardial left ventricular pacing lead.

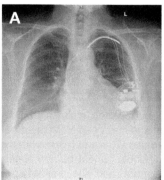
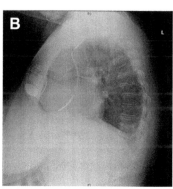

Fig. 3. Physician Assistant (PA) and lateral chest X-rays displaying downward migration of the pulse generator with lead migration.

2. Conduction system pacing: This involves leveraging the heart's intrinsic conduction system. The typical techniques include:
   a. His bundle pacing (HBP): Direct stimulation of bundle of His.
   b. Left bundle branch area pacing (LBBAP): Targets His Purkinje fibers in the left bundle branch region.

Historically, CRT has been the recommended treatment for patients with HF, specifically for patients with an EF of ≤35%, LBBB, QRS greater than 150 millisecond, and NYHA II–IV functional status treated with GDMT. Landmark trials, such as MIRACLE, COMPANION, and CARE-HF, as well as subsequent meta-analyses, have validated that these HF populations derive maximum benefit from CRT, including improvement in symptoms, decreased hospitalizations, and improved mortality.[3–7]

However, emerging evidence has illuminated the comparable advantages of CSP, either through HBP or LBBAP, for similar patient groups.[8–10] The His-Alternative trial stands out, having randomized symptomatic HF patients with LBBB to either HBP or CRT arms. The results demonstrated that HBP arm had comparable symptom alleviation and echocardiographic improvements, especially when left bundle branch block was corrected through HBP. The sample size for this study was small, however, and the HBP arm had higher pacing thresholds.[11] In fact, elevated pacing thresholds and problems with sensing can develop with HBP. The location of the His bundle at the crest of the interventricular septum can sometimes result in difficulties with adequate lead postioning.[12]

An alternative option that can achieve similar LV resynchronization is pacing distal to the bundle of His, deep within the proximal interventricular septum along the course of the left bundle branch. The LBBAP Collaborative Study Group multicenter cohort study reported 385 patients who received LBBAP pacing and demonstrated good clinical and echocardiographic outcomes at 6 months.[13] Smaller scale studies have also endorsed the benefits of LBBAP in HF patients, including one pilot study of 40 patients randomized to LBBAP or CRT showing greater improvements in LVEF with similar functional improvements in the LBBAP arm.[10] To date, there are no large randomized clinical trials demonstrating efficacy of CSP in patients with systolic HF and wide QRS. The most recent Heart Rhythm Society (HRS) guidelines list CSP as a viable alternative for cases where optimal CRT is untenable due to challenges in placing the left ventricular/CS lead.[14]

Troubleshooting

In the case detailed above, when the patient presented to the clinic with a narrow QRS but elevated left ventricular lead pacing thresholds, the necessary troubleshooting steps were executed. Generally, challenges with CIEDs can be categorized into four primary areas: pacing abnormalities, rhythm abnormalities resulting in multiple ICD shocks, inability to effectively treat VT/VF because of poor defibrillation thresholds, or poor detection.[15–17] To discern the root of the problem, both a comprehensive review of the patient's clinical history and an in-depth physical examination are essential. Using tools such as a 12-lead ECG, device memory interrogation, online telemetry, and radiographic imaging can further clarify the etiology of device dysfunction.

When evaluating the patient's history, it is vital to consider elements like previous arrhythmias, the use of antiarrhythmic drugs, etiology of HF, presence or absence of HF symptoms, palpitations, angina, and activities leading up to the CIED. Although not all these factors may be relevant for every type of malfunction, they may help rule out certain issues. During the physical examination, it is imperative to observe if certain postures exacerbate symptoms or cause shocks. Simultaneous monitoring with the use of a magnet to disable tachyarrhythmia detection and shock delivery should also be used. Concurrent use of 12-lead ECG, telemetry, and device memory can offer information on the current rhythm, battery status, pacing and sensing impedances, and irregularities in rhythm timing, which could all prove to be beneficial in troubleshooting these devices. Last, radiography with a chest X-ray can reveal lead malposition, fracture, or dislodgment. When available, these X-rays can be compared with the immediate post-implant images to assess for any discrepancies.

In this case, although the ECG, telemetry, and device interrogation provided some insights, the root cause was not uncovered until the chest X-ray was analyzed. Of note, despite the disruption in her CRT due to LV lead migration, she remained asymptomatic and without signs of ventricular dyssynchrony. The unintentional right bundle branch pacing that narrowed her QRS might have played a role in her continued well-being. Although it is challenging to pinpoint the exact reason for her lack of symptoms, several factors could have contributed including tighter GDMT management and improved MR. Nevertheless, the correction of her QRS and RBBB with the RV lead pacing her bundle cannot be completely disregarded. Furthermore, had she presented to the clinic today as a new patient, she likely wouldn't qualify for the CRT device she received 11 years ago, given the evolving criteria for CRT in HFrEF.

Device Follow-Up

The HRS/European heart rhythm association (EHRA)/Asian pacific heart rhythm society (APHRS)/Latin american heart rhythm society (LAHRS) released an expert consensus report in 2023, establishing that RM should become the standard of care for devices with this capability, and it should be made available to all patients.[18,19] Although there was an evident shift in the recommendations from various authorities, the actual transition in clinical practices and patient acceptance became prominent during the COVID-19 pandemic. With the increasing global accessibility of these devices, there arises an urgent need for an established infrastructure to manage them. Sole reliance on annual or calendar-based follow-ups, even if conducted remotely, will likely become untenable, even with substantial support staff.

To address this, the British Heart Rhythm Society (BHRS) promotes a transition to alert-based RM.[20] In this model, patients with devices capable of continuous monitoring send alerts to device clinics. These alerts are addressed based on the order they are received, rendering routine in-office or online follow-ups unnecessary. Although some patients may still prefer periodic in-person consultations, the prevailing belief is that these should not be mandatory for all CIED patients.

The HRS consensus report concurs, suggesting that alert-based RM with continuous connectivity can extend intervals between in-office check-ups, alleviating the pressure on care teams overseeing these devices. For devices on continuous RM without recent alerts, consensus deems it appropriate to have in-person visits every 24 months. For those devices without continuous connectivity, the recommendation is for remote transmissions every 3 to 12 months for pacemakers and 3 to 6 months for ICDs. As battery replacement nears due to depletion, the frequency should increase to 1 to 3 months.

Alert settings should be tailored to each patient and their respective device. High priority, or "red alerts," should be addressed within one business day. In contrast, yellow alerts typically lack the same urgency and can be dealt with in a less emergent manner. For the sake of efficiency and to minimize unnecessary notifications, nonactionable alerts for stable patients should be deactivated.

The follow-up recommendations, adapted from the HRS consensus report and BHRS, offer a structure to manage the growing prevalence of CIEDs effectively. In the case of our patient, a more intensive monitoring approach was adopted due to battery depletion and issues with the pacemaker leads. After the battery replacement, RM can be used, allowing for more extended intervals between visits, provided no complications emerge.

SUMMARY

A patient with a prior CRT-D implant at a different institution, who was lost to follow-up, presented for device interrogation. The resulting anomalous readings prompted device troubleshooting, which disclosed a displacement of the pulse generator and its leads. Intriguingly, even with these findings, the patient maintained an atrial-sensed, ventricular-paced rhythm, exhibiting a narrow QRS on the ECG, despite an underlying RBBB. This raised the possibility that the RV lead was positioned along the right bundle, thus correcting the ECG morphology. Such unintended CSP could have contributed to the patient's ongoing health, especially in the absence of effective CRT via BiV pacing. Conventionally, CRT is used for patients with ventricular asynchrony, primarily those with symptomatic HFrEF, significantly reduced EF, an inherent left bundle branch block (LBBB), and a broad QRS. Recently, alternatives to CRT, such as CSP, have gained traction and are now advocated in scenarios where traditional CRT is not feasible. For individuals equipped with these and other CIEDs, diligent troubleshooting and regular follow-up are imperative. Troubleshooting should incorporate patient history, physical examination, ECG analysis, telemetry, device interrogation, and radiographic studies. Additional tests can be pursued if initial evaluations are inconclusive. For ongoing care, it is vital for device clinics and care teams to proactively offer and leverage RM, paired with an alert-based follow-up approach, to mitigate the strain on the health care infrastructure.

CLINICS CARE POINTS

- Cardiac resynchronization therapy (CRT) is recommended for all heart failure with reduced ejection fraction (HFrEF) patients with EF of ≤35%, LBBB, QRS greater than 150 millisecond, and NYHA II–IV functional status treated with guideline-directed medical therapy (GDMT).

- Conduction system pacing with His bundle pacing or left bundle branch area pacing is reasonable for HFrEF patients with EF of ≤35%, LBBB,

QRS greater than 150 millisecond, and NYHA II–IV functional status treated with GDMT who cannot achieve effective CRT.

- Patients with cardiac implantable electronic devices should be monitored via remote monitoring to reduce clinic burden of regularly timed visits.
- Frequency of in-person visits should depend on patient's clinical status and symptom history, alarm frequency, device malfunction history, and battery life.
- Troubleshooting CIEDs during device interrogation should include 12-lead ECG, radiographs, telemetry, and patient history.

DISCLOSURE

No disclosures to report.

REFERENCES

1. Akinyele B, Marine JE, Love C, et al. Unregulated online sales of cardiac implantable electronic devices in the United States: a six-month assessment. Heart Rhythm O2 2020;1(4):235–8.
2. Writing Committee Members, ACC/AHA Joint Committee Members. 2022 AHA/ACC/HFSA guideline for the management of heart failure. J Card Fail 2022;28(5):e1–167. https://doi.org/10.1016/j.cardfail.2022.02.010.
3. Cleland JG, Daubert JC, Erdmann E, et al. The effect of cardiac resynchronization on morbidity and mortality in heart failure. N Engl J Med 2005;352(15):1539–49.
4. Bristow MR, Saxon LA, Boehmer J, et al. Cardiac-resynchronization therapy with or without an implantable defibrillator in advanced chronic heart failure. N Engl J Med 2004;350(21):2140–50.
5. Abraham WT, Fisher WG, Smith AL, et al. Cardiac resynchronization in chronic heart failure. N Engl J Med 2002;346(24):1845–53.
6. Young JB, Abraham WT, Smith AL, et al. Combined cardiac resynchronization and implantable cardioversion defibrillation in advanced chronic heart failurethe MIRACLE ICD trial. JAMA 2003;289(20):2685–94.
7. Cleland JG, Abraham WT, Linde C, et al. An individual patient meta-analysis of five randomized trials assessing the effects of cardiac resynchronization therapy on morbidity and mortality in patients with symptomatic heart failure. Eur Heart J 2013;34(46):3547–56.
8. Ponnusamy SS, Vijayaraman P. Left bundle branch block-induced cardiomyopathy: insights from left bundle branch pacing. JACC Clin Electrophysiol 2021;7(9):1155–65.
9. Sharma PS, Dandamudi G, Herweg B, et al. Permanent His-bundle pacing as an alternative to biventricular pacing for cardiac resynchronization therapy: a multicenter experience. Heart Rhythm 2018;15(3):413–20.
10. Vijayaraman P, Ponnusamy S, Cano Ó, et al. Left bundle branch area pacing for cardiac resynchronization therapy: results from the international LBBAP collaborative study group. JACC Clin Electrophysiol 2021;7(2):135–47.
11. Vinther M, Risum N, Svendsen JH, et al. A randomized trial of his pacing versus biventricular pacing in symptomatic HF patients with left bundle branch block (his-alternative). JACC Clin Electrophysiol 2021;7(11):1422–32.
12. Nagarajan VD, Ho SY, Ernst S. Anatomical considerations for his bundle pacing. Circ Arrhythm Electrophysiol 2019;12(7):e006897.
13. Yuan Z, Cheng L, Wu Y. Meta-analysis comparing safety and efficacy of left bundle branch area pacing versus his bundle pacing. Am J Cardiol 2022;164:64–72.
14. Chung MK, Patton KK, Lau CP, et al. 2023 HRS/APHRS/LAHRS guideline on cardiac physiologic pacing for the avoidance and mitigation of heart failure. Heart Rhythm 2023;20(9):e17–91.
15. Swerdlow CD, Asirvatham SJ, Ellenbogen KA, et al. Troubleshooting implantable cardioverter-defibrillator sensing problems II. Circ Arrhythm Electrophysiol 2015;8(1):212–20.
16. Swerdlow CD, Asirvatham SJ, Ellenbogen KA, et al. Troubleshooting implanted cardioverter defibrillator sensing problems I. Circ Arrhythm Electrophysiol 2014;7(6):1237–61.
17. Saeed M. Troubleshooting implantable cardioverter-defibrillators: an overview for physicians who are not electrophysiologists. Tex Heart Inst J 2011;38(4):355–7.
18. Ferrick AM, Raj SR, Deneke T, et al. 2023 HRS/EHRA/APHRS/LAHRS expert consensus statement on practical management of the remote device clinic. Europace 2023;25(5). https://doi.org/10.1093/europace/euad123.
19. Kusumoto FM, Schoenfeld MH, Wilkoff BL, et al. 2017 HRS expert consensus statement on cardiovascular implantable electronic device lead management and extraction. Heart Rhythm 2017;14(12):e503–51.
20. Roberts E, Wright I, Slade A, et al. Clinical standards and guidelines for the follow up of cardiac implantable electronic devices (CIEDs) for cardiac rhythm management. 2022. Available at: https://bhrs.com/wp-content/uploads/2022/06/BHRS-CIED-FU-Standards-June22.pdf.

Atrial Tachycardia Masquerading as Atrial Fibrillation Following Bi-Atrial MAZE Procedure

Fengwei Zou, MD, Andrew Krumerman, MD*

KEYWORDS

- Atrial fibrillation • Atrial tachycardia • Premtaure atrial contractions (PACs) • Catheter ablation
- MAZE procedure

KEY POINTS

- Recurrent atrial arrhythmia following surgical MAZE procedure is often difficult to diagnose due to low-voltage atrial activity on electrocardiogram and tendency to masquerade as atrial fibrillation (AF).
- Catheter ablation of patients with recurrent arrhythmia following surgical MAZE procedure requires careful mapping to elucidate areas of scar surrounding the sinus and atrioventricular nodal regions.
- Premature atrial contractions are associated with a higher risk of incident AF and stroke.

INTRODUCTION

Atrial fibrillation (AF) is one of the most common supraventricular arrhythmias associated with mitral valve (MV) diseases.[1] Both endocardial catheter ablation and surgical Cox-MAZE procedures are effective rhythm control interventions to restore and maintain sinus rhythm in patients with valvular AF. In the 2017 HRS/EHRA/ECAS/APHRS/SOLAECE expert consensus statement on catheter and surgical ablation of AF, surgical Cox MAZE procedure received a Class I indication in patients undergoing concomitant open atrial surgeries such as MV repair or replacement.[2] Despite the efficacy in maintaining electrical isolation within its box lesions, surgical Cox-MAZE procedures are associated with atrial scarring and complex atrial tachycardias (ATs) originating near the surgical lesions. Here, the authors present a case of a young woman undergoing repeat AT ablation after a cryoMAZE procedure during concomitant bioprosthetic MV replacement and the challenges in distinguishing AT from AF due to the lack of identifiable P waves on surface electrocardiogram (ECG) from diffuse bi-atrial scarring. This case illustrates pitfalls associated with the surgical MAZE procedure and highlights the challenges in postoperative atrial arrhythmias diagnosis and management.

CASE PRESENTATION

A 34-year-old female patient without past medical history presented to the emergency room with increasing intermittent chest pain, palpitation, dizziness, and shortness of breath for the past 6 months. She was found to have redundant MV with anterior leaflet prolapse causing severe mitral regurgitation on transthoracic echocardiogram and paroxysmal AF on telemetry likely secondary to the MV disease. She was referred to cardiothoracic surgery and underwent bioprosthetic MV replacement, tricuspid valve (TV) repair, left atrial appendage (LAA) surgical excision with AtriCure

Montefiore-Einstein Center for Heart and Vascular Care, Montefiore Medical Center, 111 East 210th Street, Bronx, NY 10467, USA
* Corresponding author. Montefiore Center for Heart & Vascular DIsease, 111 E 210 Street, Bronx, NY 10467.
E-mail address: akrumerm@montefiore.org

Card Electrophysiol Clin 16 (2024) 169–174
https://doi.org/10.1016/j.ccep.2023.10.004
1877-9182/24/© 2023 Elsevier Inc. All rights reserved.

Clip, and bi-atrial cryoMAZE procedure. Her postoperative course was complicated by inferior wall myocardial infarction necessitating percutaneous coronary intervention of the right posterior descending coronary artery and recurrent frequent palpitations for which she was referred back to the arrhythmia service. A 12-lead ECG demonstrated periods of regularity and irregularity representing either atrial flutter with low-amplitude flutter waves, sinus rhythm with low-amplitude P waves, or junctional rhythm (**Fig. 1**A). She was started on verapamil 120 mg daily and placed on 14-day Ziopatch, which showed AF with controlled ventricular rate (see **Fig. 1**B). Patient continued to have symptoms despite medical therapy and was started on oral anticoagulation (OAC) in preparation for catheter ablation. Unfortunately, she suffered from severe menstrual bleeding while on

OAC with her serum hemoglobin nearly halved before ablation. She received transfusions and was brought back on half-dose OAC a few months later after recovery.

At the time of electrophysiological study, the underlying rhythm was sinus bradycardia with frequent premature atrial contractions (PACs) with earliest PAC atrial activation noted at the distal coronary sinus (CS) electrodes (**Fig. 2**A). Intracardiac electroanatomical mapping (EAM) revealed diffuse scarring of both atria. Electrical connections were absent in all pulmonary veins and along the posterior wall consistent with an intact MAZE box lesion set. Voltage mapping revealed low voltage throughout the right atrium except for an area along the lateral wall spanning from superior vena cava (SVC) to inferior vena cava and a small area along the interatrial septum.

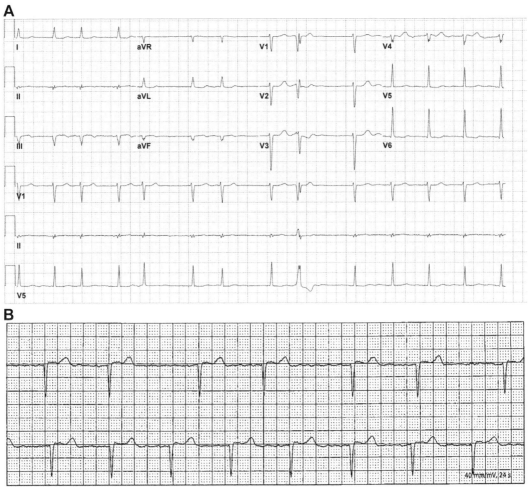

Fig. 1. Postoperative 12-lead ECG in the arrhythmia clinic and Ziopatch rhythm strip. (*A*) The underlying rhythm is likely AF with no visible P waves but periods of regularity and irregularity representing either atrial flutter with low-amplitude flutter waves, sinus rhythm with low-amplitude P waves, or junctional rhythm. (*B*) Ziopatch rhythm strip showing AF with controlled ventricular rate.

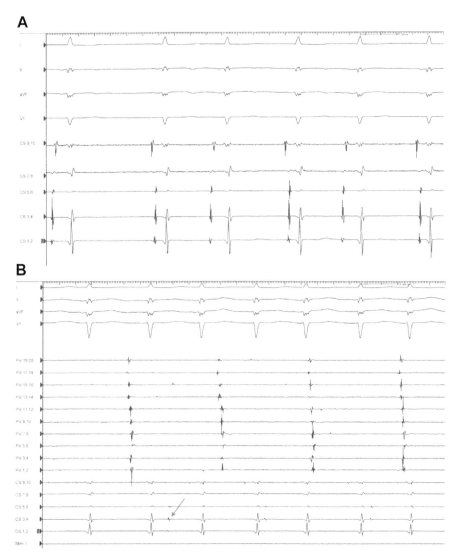

Fig. 2. Intracardiac EGMs during catheter ablation. (*A*) Surface ECG with an irregularly irregular rhythm. Coronary sinus electrograms demonstrate sinus rhythm with frequent APCs. (*B*) Surface ECG and intracardiac electrograms from PentaRay (PV 1–20) and coronary sinus catheters (CS 1–10). The PentaRay catheter is positioned along the posterior left atrial wall and demonstrates dissociated potentials consistent with an intact MAZE box lesion. The blue arrow demonstrates dissociated potentials from the coronary sinus following RF ablation of atrial tachycardia originating from the anterolateral mitral annulus.

Atrial pacing from the SVC-RA junction demonstrated 1:1 atrioventricular (AV) conduction at 600 millisecond and a stim-to-QRS duration of 300 millisecond. Isoproterenol infusion elicited frequent left-sided unifocal PACs mapped to the anterolateral mitral annulus. Radiofrequency application to this site eliminated PACs and resulted in electrical isolation of the CS (see **Fig. 2**B). The patient was discharged home, and verapamil was discontinued. However, 1 year after ablation, she again reported fatigue and dyspnea on exertion, and her personal wearable device recorded an irregularly irregular rhythm at the rate of 90 to

100 bpm. Her verapamil was restarted and repeat Ziopatch showed 100% atrial flutter with controlled ventricular rate. She was started on dronedarone 400 mg bid for pharmacologic rhythm control. Despite these efforts, she remained symptomatic and returned for EPS.

This time, EAM (**Fig. 3**) again demonstrated complete electrical isolation in all pulmonary veins, the posterior wall, and the entire left atrium including the distal CS. A small area of low-voltage EGMs were recorded along the interatrial septum. Isoproterenol administration revealed non-pulmonary vein triggers originating in the right

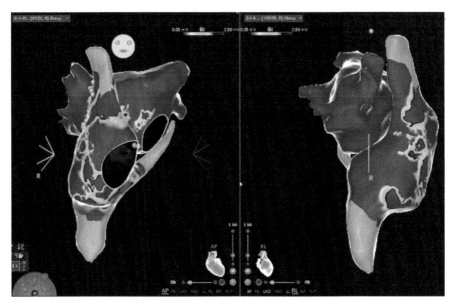

Fig. 3. Electroanatomical map of the atria. Voltage map demonstrating extensive scar with a strip of tissue along the lateral aspect of the right atrium (RA) demonstrating normal voltage. Another area where conduction was preserved was along the septum where the AV node/His bundle were located. This area had fractionated electrograms and low- to moderate-voltage EGMs. Voltage scale = 0.05 to 0.5 mV.

atrium. A baseline voltage map of the right atrium revealed extensive scar with a strip of tissue along the lateral aspect demonstrating normal voltage. Another area where conduction was preserved was along the septum where the AV node/His bundle were located. This area had fractionated electrograms and low- to moderate-voltage EGMs. Isoproterenol infusion revealed frequent PACs that were mapped to the superior lateral right atrium. RF energy applied to this area resulted in the elimination of PACs. Repeat challenge with isoproterenol-induced frequent PACs, originating from the anterior septum just posterior to the His bundle electrogram. As this area represented the only conduction pathway between the atria and the AV node, no ablation was performed. EPS also revealed prolonged AH interval of 350 millisecond and prolonged sinus node recovery time with a secondary pause (**Fig. 4**). Based on these findings, dual-chamber pacemaker was subsequently implanted. The patient tolerated the procedure well and was discharged home without anticoagulation.

DISCUSSION

Concomitant Cox MAZE procedure during open atrial surgery is an effective approach to restore sinus rhythm in patients with AF and valvular disease needing open heart surgery. Meta-analysis of randomized controlled trials reported 12-month freedom from atrial arrhythmias from 60% to 90% after cardiac surgery and concomitant surgical ablation without significantly increased safety events.[3] The modern Cox MAZE procedure has evolved from the traditional cut-and-sew approach to radiofrequency- or cryoenergy-based surgical ablation, which most likely explains the wide range of effectiveness reported across these trials. Small-sample electrophysiological studies in patients with atrial arrhythmia recurrence after Cox MAZE suggested that the cut-and-sew approach is more likely to keep the pulmonary veins durably isolated compared with other approaches.[4] More often than not, post-MAZE atrial arrhythmias present as non-AF atrial arrhythmias such as focal ATs and incisional atrial flutters.[5] However, the diagnosis of atrial arrhythmias from surface ECG or telemetry monitoring is often challenging due to low atrial voltage and low-amplitude P waves from extensive atrial scarring after MAZE.

In this case, the initial diagnosis of atrial arrhythmia was believed to be AF due to the irregularly irregular-appearing ventricular rhythm on continuous ECG monitoring. It was not until the patient was brought for invasive EPS that the diagnosis of sinus rhythm with frequent APCs was made. Ultimately, electrical isolation of the pulmonary veins and posterior wall was confirmed and the diagnosis of AT was achieved. Early and accurate diagnosis of the correct atrial arrhythmia is important not only for choosing the optimal management strategy and potential pharmacologic agents but also for deciding whether systemic

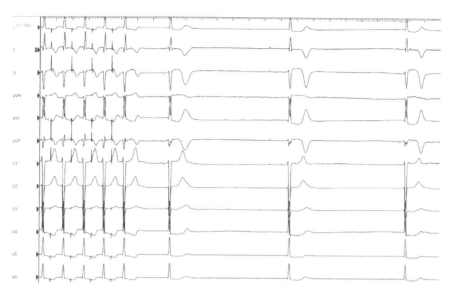

Fig. 4. Sinus node recovery time. A 12-lead ECG demonstrating a prolonged secondary pause following pacing at 500 millisecond for 15 seconds.

anticoagulation is indicated. In this young female patient of reproductive age, the initiation of systemic OAC in anticipation of AF ablation led to a significant and life-threatening bleeding event that simply could not be overlooked. The benefit of LAA ligation during the open heart surgery can mitigate the use of systemic anticoagulation in this patient and others at risk of major bleeding. On the flip side of the coin, studies have shown that frequent PACs are not only a predictor of developing AF but also a predictor of stroke risk without AF.[6,7] Dichotomized analysis of frequent PACs has been associated with ~3-fold risk of developing AF and ~2.5-fold risk of developing stroke.[7] Whether or not systemic OAC is indicated for such patients remains contentious and is currently not reflected in current guidelines. This patient was eventually discharged home without systemic anticoagulation due to her previous LAA ligation and history of severe bleeding.

Another key point worth noting in this case is that although cryoMAZE achieved durable pulmonary vein and posterior wall isolation confirmed by EAM, extensive scarring in both atria was present. This scarring resulted in delayed conduction from the sinus node to the AV node. Prolongation of the AH interval due to prolonged right atrial conduction time results in pseudo-block.[8] In the aforementioned case, only a narrow corridor of tissue with normal conduction was noted, which can complicate the ablation of incisional arrhythmias. Careful mapping of both atria was required to avoid injury to the native conduction system as well as tracts of tissue that lie between the sinoatrial and AV

nodes. In this case, preoperative discussions with shared decision-making played a key role in allowing the operator to target non-pulmonary vein triggers in the right atrium. The patient understood that there was a high likelihood that right atrium (RA) ablation would result in the need for pacemaker therapy.

SUMMARY

Evaluation of patients with recurrent arrhythmia following surgical MAZE is often challenging due to low voltage in both atria. Patients with low atrial voltage and low-amplitude P waves on ECG often are diagnosed with AF in settings where frequent APCs are noted, complicating the decision of systemic anticoagulation and pharmacologic antiarrhythmic agents. Catheter ablation of patients with recurrent arrhythmia following surgical MAZE procedure requires careful mapping to elucidate area of scar surrounding the sinus and AV nodal regions.

CLINICS CARE POINTS

- Recurrent arrhythmia following surgical MAZE procedure can be challenging to diagnose and treat.
- Diffuse scarring of the atria makes atrial activity difficult to discern on 12-lead electrocardiogram.
- Sinus rhythm with frequent APCs can masquerade as atrial fibrillation.

- Atrial catheter ablation postsurgical MAZE procedure can result in sinus node exit block or pseudo-atrial fibrillation block.
- Careful preoperative planning and shared decision-making are necessary when considering electrophysiologic study with ablation in such patients.

DISCLOSURES

No disclosures to report.

REFERENCES

1. Kubala M, de Chillou C, Bohbot Y, et al. Arrhythmias in patients with valvular heart disease: gaps in knowledge and the way forward. Front Cardiovasc Med 2022;9:792559.
2. Calkins H, Hindricks G, Cappato R, et al. HRS/EHRA/ECAS/APHRS/SOLAECE expert consensus statement on catheter and surgical ablation of atrial fibrillation. Heart Rhythm 2017;14(10):e275–444.
3. Phan K, Xie A, La Meir M, et al. Surgical ablation for treatment of atrial fibrillation in cardiac surgery: a cumulative meta-analysis of randomised controlled trials. Heart 2014;100(9):722–30.
4. Winkle RA, Fleming W, Mead RH, et al. Catheter ablation for failed surgical maze: comparison of cut and sew vs. non-cut and sew maze. J Interv Card Electrophysiol 2019;55(2):183–9.
5. Wazni OM, Saliba W, Fahmy T, et al. Atrial arrhythmias after surgical maze: findings during catheter ablation. J Am Coll Cardiol 2006;48(7):1405–9.
6. Farinha JM, Gupta D, Lip GYH. Frequent premature atrial contractions as a signalling marker of atrial cardiomyopathy, incident atrial fibrillation, and stroke. Cardiovasc Res 2023;119(2):429–39.
7. Himmelreich JCL, Lucassen WAM, Heugen M, et al. Frequent premature atrial contractions are associated with atrial fibrillation, brain ischaemia, and mortality: a systematic review and meta-analysis. Europace 2019;21(5):698–707.
8. Do U, Nam GB, Kim M, et al. Inter/intra-atrial dissociation in patients with maze procedure and its clinical implications: pseudo-block and pseudo-ventricular tachycardia. J Am Heart Assoc 2020;9(23):e018241.

Arrhythmias of the Left Atrial Appendage

Approaches to the Definitive Management of Atrial Tachycardia from the LAA Stump

Xiaodong Zhang, MD, PhD[a], Sujoy Khasnavis, MD[b], Samer Saouma, MD[a],
Luigi Di Biase, MD, PhD[a],*

KEYWORDS

• Atrial tachycardia • Left atrial appendage • Stump isolation • AtriClip

KEY POINTS

- Residual appendageal stumps are often present post surgical exclusion of Left atrial appendage (LAA).
- Atrial tachycardia can originate from LAA stump.
- Proximal isolation of the LAA stump can induce remission of LAA-driven arrhythmias.

 Video content accompanies this article at http://www.cardiacep.theclinics.com.

INTRODUCTION

As the leading form of cardiac arrhythmia across the world, atrial fibrillation (AF) is projected to affect millions of people in the coming decades.[1] The left atrial appendage (LAA) has been shown to be an important trigger of AF in patients with persistent and long-standing persistent AF.[2] The LAA, previously considered a vestigial structure, is now recognized as a significant contributor to arrhythmia and thromboembolism in patients with a history of AF.[3] Stasis of blood in the LAA leads to thrombus formation and has been identified as a source of embolic stroke in nearly 90% of cases of AF.[4] Although anticoagulation therapy has been effective in stroke prevention, patients at increased risk of bleeding, who are intolerant to warfarin or direct oral anticoagulants, require consideration of alternative therapies for stroke prevention. These therapies include LAA exclusion via surgical amputation or complete obliteration of the appendage with clips and other occlusion devices.[5] Moreover, thoracoscopic exclusion of the LAA is made possible with the AtriClip device (AtriCure, OH, USA), often accompanied by an epicardial surgical ablation.[6,7] Because of variations in anatomy and approach, residual appendageal stumps are often present postprocedure and thought to be a source of sustained arrhythmia and thromboembolism.[8–10] We describe the case of a 65-year-old male patient with a history of AtriClip LAA exclusion, who had recurrent AF and atrial tachycardia (AT) despite multiple ablation procedures. After undergoing ablation and isolation of the LAA stump, he had complete resolution of his arrhythmias.

CLINICAL SCENARIO

The patient is a 65-year-old man with a history of colon cancer, diabetes mellitus, hypertension, obstructive sleep apnea, and long-standing persistent AF. He is status-post pulmonary vein isolation (PVI) and cavo-tricuspid isthmus ablation

[a] Montefiore Medical Center, Albert Einstein College of Medicine, Bronx, NY 10467, USA; [b] Jacobi Medical Center, Albert Einstein College of Medicine, Bronx, NY 10461, USA
* Corresponding author.
E-mail address: ldibiase@montefiore.org

Card Electrophysiol Clin 16 (2024) 175–180
https://doi.org/10.1016/j.ccep.2023.10.018

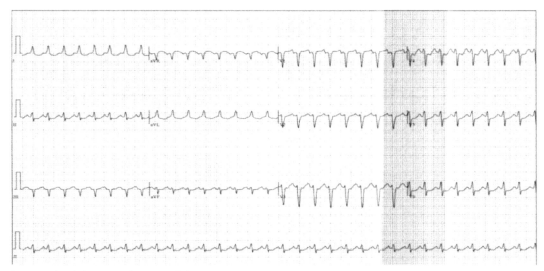

Fig. 1. 12-lead electrocardiogram of the patient's recurrent AT.

in 2009. In 2012, he developed recurrent AF, so he underwent a repeat ablation, where pulmonary veins were reisolated, and a mitral isthmus line was created, and bidirectional block was achieved. He later underwent an epicardial ablation for recurrent AF, along with clipping of the LAA by AtriClip in 2017. Then, he developed recurrent Tikosyn-refractory paroxysmal atrial arrhythmias prompting multiple visits to the emergency department (**Fig. 1**). Sinus rhythm was restored with multiple direct current cardioversions before the patient presented to our institution in March 2023 for an electrophysiology study and catheter ablation. His medications included Eliquis 5 mg twice daily, metoprolol succinate 25 mg once daily, and dofetilide 250 mcg twice daily. A transthoracic echocardiogram showed a normal left ventricular ejection fraction (60%–65%), mild left atrial enlargement, normal right ventricular size

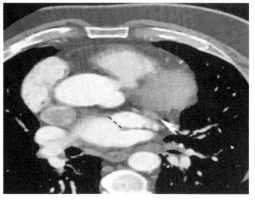

Fig. 2. CT scan showing the LAA clip (blue *arrow*) distal to the LAA ostium (dashed black *line*).

and function, and absence of any significant valvular disease. A preprocedural computed tomography (CT) scan revealed 2 separate left pulmonary veins, 2 separate right pulmonary veins, and a distally applied LAA clip with a remnant LAA stump free of thrombus (**Fig. 2**).

ELECTROPHYSIOLOGY STUDY AND CATHETER ABLATION

The patient arrived at the electrophysiology laboratory in normal sinus rhythm. Dual transeptal access was obtained under intracardiac echocardiography and fluoroscopy guidance. A multipolar high-density mapping catheter (Octaray, Biosense Webster, CA, USA) was used to build an electroanatomic map of the left atrium. The initial voltage map revealed a severely scarred left atrium, electrically silent pulmonary veins and posterior wall, and conduction block across the posterior mitral isthmus. During catheter manipulation close to the LAA, an AT with a cycle length of 400 milliseconds and 1:1 atrioventricular relationship was induced, similar to the patient's clinical tachycardia. Local activation time (LAT) mapping revealed a microreentrant AT originating from the base of the LAA (**Fig. 3**; Video 1). Radiofrequency energy was applied at the site of earliest activation exhibiting a long fractionated electrogram leading to slowing and eventual termination of the tachycardia (**Fig. 4**; Video 2). A decision was made to electrically isolate the LAA stump. Interestingly, while isolating the LAA, we observed separate isolation of the anterior lobe of LAA with dissociated firing (**Fig. 5**). Anterior and posterior lobes were both isolated and confirmed by evidence of dissociated potentials (**Fig. 6**). High-dose isoproterenol (20 mcg/

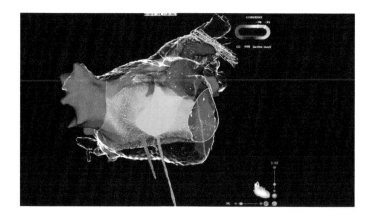

Fig. 3. Activation map of the AT originating from the base of the LAA stump with superimposed CT scan showing the location of AtriClip.

min) was infused and programmed electrical stimulation was delivered without induction of atrial arrhythmia. The patient tolerated the procedure well and had an uncomplicated postoperative course. Dofetilide was discontinued and he was discharged home the next day in sinus rhythm. At 2-month follow-up, he remained in sinus rhythm, reported feeling well, and denied palpitations or shortness of breath.

DISCUSSION

LAA exclusion is a viable therapy that is increasingly being used to reduce thromboembolic risk in patients with AF intolerant to anticoagulation.

Endocardial and epicardial approaches and various tools and devices have been used to achieve complete LAA exclusion. Devices delivered through the endocardial approach, including Watchman (Boston Scientific, MA, USA) and Amplatzer Amulet (Abbott, CA, USA), have been widely adopted.[11] Surgical exclusion of the LAA has been achieved through myriad techniques with variable success rates. These are often performed at the time of cardiothoracic surgery and include suture ligation, surgical excision with suture closure, and stapling of LAA without excision. Studies have shown low success rates and have often led to incomplete occlusion with residual leaks that can paradoxically increase the risk of

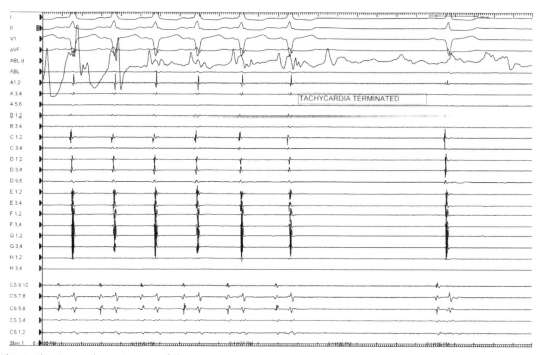

Fig. 4. Slowing and termination of the AT.

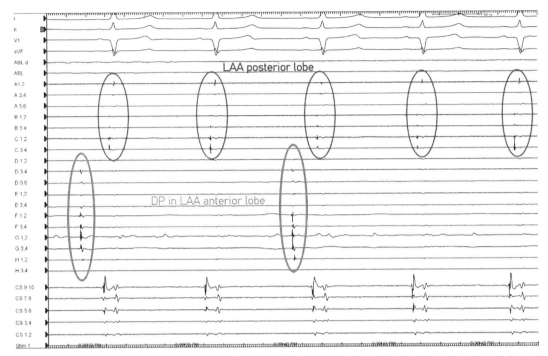

Fig. 5. Multipolar catheter in the appendage: Splines A–C in the posterior lobe with signals (red circle) and D–H in the anterior lobe with evidence of dissociated potentials (blue circle).

thrombus formation.[5] AtriClip has emerged as a novel epicardial device that can achieve LAA exclusion by applying a clip to the base of the LAA. An added advantage to this device is the option to be delivered through a thoracoscopic approach, without the need for a sternotomy. In fact, similar to our patient's case, the AtriClip is now being introduced as an essential part of the hybrid convergent ablation procedure. Initial studies have shown high success rates of AtriClip in achieving complete LAA exclusion.[8] However, cases of incomplete occlusions or persistent LAA

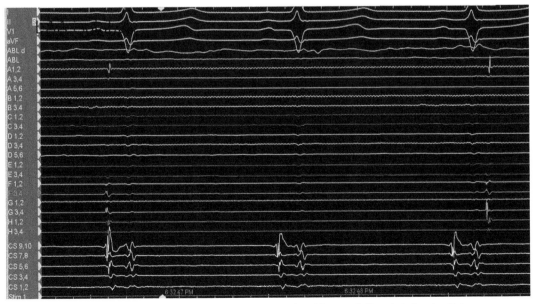

Fig. 6. Multipolar catheter inside the isolated LAA stump with evidence of dissociated potentials.

stump have been reported. Recent data show that AtriClip placement has been associated with residual stump rate incidence of 46.2%, with 19% incidence of stumps greater than 10 mm.[12] Furthermore, studies have shown that the presence of a residual stump posed a thrombogenic and arrhythmogenic risk, and isolation of the stump is associated with arrhythmia-free survival.[13,14] This adds to the existing data that show that LAA isolation is associated with less AF/AT recurrence. Alkhouli and colleagues reported on the findings of various clinical trials such as BELIEF, which described a 1-year recurrence rate for AF that was 2-fold lower in patients who underwent LAA electrical isolation and standard PVI as compared with patients who underwent standard PVI alone.[15] Lakkireddy and colleagues reported registry data demonstrating that during a 1-year follow-up course, epicardial LAA ligation led to a 26% improvement in the rate of AF/AT recurrence as compared with standard ablation alone.[16] Romero and colleagues found in their prospective study that during a 5-year follow-up period, freedom from recurrent AT and AF without antiarrhythmic agents was nearly 20% greater in the patient group with LAA isolation and standard ablation as compared with the patient group with standard ablation alone.[17] Finally, the rate and likelihood of arrhythmogenic and thromboembolic events following surgical LAA exclusion warrants further studies given the association between the presence and size of the stump and thromboembolic complications and arrhythmia recurrence.[12,14]

SUMMARY

In summary, LAA is becoming a widely recognized source of atrial arrhythmia and thromboembolism in patients with AF. Epicardial LAA exclusion procedures such as AtriClip have evolved as an adjunct to various cardiac surgeries in patients with AF, especially in those with high bleeding risk. It has been shown that the location of appendage exclusion and size of the residual LAA stump are significant contributors to atrial arrhythmias. Our case demonstrates that the proximal isolation of the LAA is more likely to induce remission of LAA-driven arrhythmias and promote the long-term maintenance of normal sinus rhythm.

CLINICS CARE POINTS

- LAA stump has an arrhythmogenic potential, in addition to the thrombogenic potential.

- Ablation of the tachycardia originating from the LAA stump can be challenging.
- LAA isolation in such cases improves arrhythmia-free survival.

DISCLOSURE

The authors have nothing to disclose.

SUPPLEMENTARY DATA

Supplementary data related to this article can be found online at https://doi.org/10.1016/j.ccep.2023.10.018.

REFERENCES

1. Morillo CA, Banerjee A, Perel P, et al. Atrial fibrillation: the current epidemic. J Geriatr Cardiol 2017; 14:195–203.
2. Di Biase L, Burkhardt JD, Mohanty P, et al. Left atrial appendage: an underrecognized trigger site of atrial fibrillation. Circulation 2010;122(2):109–18.
3. Bansal M, Kasliwal RR. Echocardiography for left atrial appendage structure and function. Indian Heart J 2012;64(5):469–75.
4. Whitlock RP, Healey JS, Connolly SJ. Left atrial appendage occlusion does not eliminate the need for warfarin. Circulation 2009;120(19):1927–32.
5. Soltesz E, Gillinov M. The left atrial appendage: a surgical target. J Thorac Cardiovasc Surg 2017; 153:1106–7.
6. Holmes DR Jr, Kar S, Price MJ, et al. Prospective randomized evaluation of the watchman left atrial appendage closure device in patients with atrial fibrillation versus long-term warfarin therapy: the PREVAIL trial [published correction appears in J Am Coll Cardiol 2014;64:1186. J Am Coll Cardiol 2014;64:1–12.
7. Lawrance CP, Henn MC, Damiano RJ Jr. Surgical ablation for atrial fibrillation: techniques, indications, and results. Curr Opin Cardiol 2015;30(1):58.
8. Ailawadi G, Gerdisch MW, Harvey RL, et al. Exclusion of the left atrial appendage with a novel device: early results of a multicenter trial. J Thorac Cardiovasc Surg 2011;142:1002–9.
9. Bedeir K, Warriner S, Kofsky E, et al. Left atrial appendage epicardial clip (AtriClip): essentials and post-procedure management. J Atr Fibrillation 2019;11:2087.
10. Aznaurov SG, Ball SK, Ellis CR. Thoracoscopic Atriclip closure of left atrial appendage after failed ligation via LARIAT. JACC Cardiovasc Interv 2015;8:e265–7.
11. Lakkireddy D, Thaler D, Ellis CR, et al. Amplatzer amulet left atrial appendage occluder versus watchman device for stroke prophylaxis (Amulet

IDE): a randomized, controlled trial. Circulation 2021;144(19):1543–52.

12. Ahmed A, Pothineni NVK, Singh V, et al. Long-term imaging and clinical outcomes of surgical left atrial appendage occlusion with atriclip. Am J Cardiol 2023;201:193–9.

13. Di Biase L, Burkhardt JD, Mohanty P, et al. Left atrial appendage isolation in patients with longstanding persistent AF undergoing catheter ablation: BELIEF trial. J Am Coll Cardiol 2016;68(18):1929–40.

14. Mohanty S, Di Biase L, Trivedi C, et al. Arrhythmogenecity and thrombogenicity of the residual left atrial appendage stump following surgical exclusion of the appendage in patients with atrial fibrillation. J Cardiovasc Electrophysiol 2019;30(3):339–47.

15. Alkhouli M, Di Biase L, Natale A, et al. Nonthrombogenic roles of the left atrial appendage: JACC review topic of the week. J Am Coll Cardiol 2023;81(11):1063–75.

16. Lakkireddy D, Sridhar Mahankali A, Kanmanthareddy A, et al. Left atrial appendage ligation and ablation for persistent atrial fibrillation: the LAALA-AF Registry. J Am Coll Cardiol EP 2015;1(3):153–60.

17. Romero J, Di Biase L, Mohanty S, et al. Longterm outcomes of left atrial appendage electrical isolation in patients with nonparoxysmal atrial fibrillation: a propensity score-matched analysis. Circ Arrhythm Electrophysiol 2020;13(11):e008390.

Bipolar Ablation for an Intramural Septal Atrial Tachycardia

Tommaso Barbati, MS[a], Vincenzo Mirco La Fazia, MD[b], Carola Gianni, MD[b], Sanghamitra Mohanty, MD[c], Andrea Natale, MD[d],*

KEYWORDS

- Atrial fibrillation ablation • Atrial tachycardia • Bipolar ablation • Radiofrequency catheter ablation
- Nonpulmonary vein triggers

KEY POINTS

- Role of extrapulmonary triggers (beyond the well-established role of pulmonary veins in atrial fibrillation, extrapulmonary triggers, especially in cases of persistent atrial fibrillation (AF) and long-standing persistent AF, have a significant contribution to recurrence).
- Challenges with septal atrial tachycardias (post-AF ablation atrial tachycardias originating from the interatrial septum [IAS] can be especially challenging due to their deep intramural location and the difficulty of achieving effective ablation with standard unipolar techniques).
- Bipolar radiofrequency catheter ablation (B-RFCA) as an alternative (in cases resistant to standard approaches, B-RFCA provides an effective alternative for terminating tachycardias that originate from deep intramural locations such as the IAS).

INTRODUCTION

Atrial fibrillation (AF) is one of the most common arrhythmias and is estimated to influence more than 10 million people in the United States alone by 2030.[1] It is well known that pulmonary veins (PVs) play an important role in the maintenance of AF.[2] Therefore, PV isolation is considered the standard of care in the treatment of AF.[2,3]

However, extrapulmonary triggers can play a significant role especially in the case of persistent AF and long-standing persistent AF (LSPAF), thus they should be considered in the treatment of AF to reduce recurrence.[4] Extrapulmonary triggers include left atrial appendage (LAA), coronary sinus (CS), posterior wall (PW), superior vena cava (SVC), and interatrial septum (IAS), with an estimated prevalence of ~70% in LSPAF.[5]

In some patients, ablation results in macro-reentrant or focal atrial tachycardias (ATs) that require a repeat ablation procedure.

The IAS has been identified to be the thickest structure of the left atrium and could be a challenging site during post-AF ablation septal ATs.[6,7]

In such situations, bipolar radiofrequency catheter ablation (B-RFCA) could be a safe and effective approach to provide the necessary advantage needed to ablate focal or reentrant forms of arrhythmia by creating transmural lesions.

Herein, we describe a case of septal focal AT resulting after AF ablation that was terminated with the use B-RFCA.

a Texas Cardiac Arrhythmia Institute, St David's Medical Center, 3000 N Interstate Hwy-35 Suite 722, Austin, TX 78705, USA; b Texas Cardiac Arrhythmia Institute, St David's Medical Center, 3000 N Interstate Hwy-35 Suite 720, Austin, TX 78705, USA; c Texas Cardiac Arrhythmia Institute, St David's Medical Center, 1015 East 32nd Street, Suite 408, Austin, TX 787059, USA; d Texas Cardiac Arrhythmia Institute, St David's Medical Center, 3000 N Interstate Hwy 35 Suite 700, Austin, TX 78705, USA
* Corresponding author.
E-mail address: dr.natale@gmail.com

Card Electrophysiol Clin 16 (2024) 181–186
https://doi.org/10.1016/j.ccep.2023.10.001
1877-9182/24/© 2023 Elsevier Inc. All rights reserved.

CASE REPORT

A 70-year-old male patient with persistent AF presented for transcatheter ablation for AF recurrence despite multiple earlier ablations. The patient had a medical history of hypertension, hyperlipidemia, coronary artery disease, and severe obstructive sleep apnea on continuous positive airway pressure. Transthoracic echocardiography showed a normal left ventricular ejection fraction (55%) and mild mitral regurgitation and tricuspid regurgitation.

He experienced AF recurrences every year since his most recent ablation in 2014, despite multiple electrical cardioversions and antiarrhythmic therapy. The patient reported being highly symptomatic from AF with fatigue, activity intolerance, dyspnea on exertion, and palpitations.

Antiarrhythmic therapy (Sotalol 120 mg twice per day) was tapered with last dose 3 days before procedure. The patient presented to the electrophysiology laboratory in AF.

The procedure was conducted under general anesthesia and uninterrupted oral anticoagulation (Apixaban 5 mg twice per day).

A 20-pole linear catheter (Biosense Webster, Diamond Bar, CA, USA) was placed with electrodes spanning from the SVC and crista terminalis (CT) to the CS. Intracardiac echocardiography (ICE; Soundstar ICE, Biosense Webster, Diamond Bar, CA, USA) was placed in the right atrium to guide transseptal puncture. A circular mapping catheter (CMC; Lasso 20 mm/10 electrodes, Biosense Webster, Irvine, CA) and an ablation catheter (QDOT MICRO, Biosense Webster, Diamond Bar, CA, USA) were advanced into left atrium for mapping and ablation, respectively. Three-dimensional electroanatomic mapping was performed with the use of the Carto 3-D mapping system (Biosense Webster, Diamond Bar, CA, USA).

All PVs remained electrically silent from the previous ablation. Despite isolation of the left atrial PW, SVC, CS, and LAA, patient remained in AF.

We placed catheters according to our standard protocol to find non-PV triggers: the CMC in the left superior PV recording the far-field LAA activity, the ablation catheter in the right superior PV that records the far-field IAS, and a 20-pole catheter with electrodes spanning from the SVC to the CS. With this catheter setup, when focal ectopic atrial activity is observed, their activation sequence is compared with that of sinus rhythm, thus leading to the identification of the area of origin.[4]

The P wave is used as the reference to identify the site of earliest activation and correlated to the timing of the local electrograms.

Because the patient was still in AF, external cardioversion with the restoration of sinus rhythm and subsequent pharmacologic challenge test with high-dose isoproterenol infusion (20 μg/min) were started in order to identify non-PV triggers responsible for AF.

Shortly after, AT with a cycle length (CL) of 250 milliseconds was induced.

Synchronous activation was documented in both the CT and CS segments of the 20-pole catheter and earlier far-field atrial activity was recorded by the ablation catheter, thus suggesting origin from the IAS area.

RF ablation was delivered along the left atrial septum resulting in the termination of AT to sinus rhythm.

Additional RF ablation lesions were placed along the left atrial septum to achieve durable lesions.

A few hours after ablation, the patient experienced recurrence of symptomatic AT with heart rate more than 140 beats/min and redo AT ablation was planned for the following day.

The patient arrived in electrophysiology laboratory in AT. Recording and activation mapping showed the same arrhythmia origin as the previous procedure.

Early tachycardia electrograms were recorded by the ablation catheter positioned on the right side of the IAS (**Fig. 1**). RF ablation energy was delivered for 44 seconds to the right atrial septum with brief termination of the tachycardia to sinus rhythm before spontaneous reinitiation of the same AT.

The Thermocool SF catheter (Biosense Webster, Diamond Bar, CA, USA) was then advanced into the left atrium. Earlier potentials were targeted for ablation along the left atrial septum with a 16-second delivery of RF energy, resulting in the prolongation of the tachycardia CL before termination of AT to sinus rhythm, which was followed by a spontaneous reinitiation of AT (**Fig. 2**).

An even earlier low voltage potential was then mapped and targeted again from the right atrium at the level of the *fossa ovalis*, leading to another brief termination of AT (**Fig. 3**).

Considering the thickness of the septum pictured on ICE and the prolonged ablation required from both sides of the septum, the decision was made to ablate using a bipolar ablation approach to create a deep transmural lesion in the IAS.

An additional Thermocool SF catheter was placed along the right atrial septum across from the spot of tachycardia termination in the left atrial septum, and RF energy was delivered from the catheter positioned in the left atrium to the one in the right atrium (**Fig. 4**).

A

B

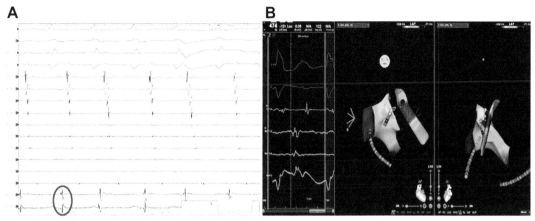

Fig. 1. (A) Intracardiac electrograms recordings before the first termination on the right side of the IAS. The red circle shows the earliest potential recorded from the ablation catheter.(B) CARTO-3D voltage map showing early potential (−151 ms) and corresponding sharp (near-field) electrograms on the right side of the IAS before the first termination in anteroposterior and left lateral views.

The bipolar energy delivery lasted 62 seconds with progressive increase in power from 20 W to 35 W, an average temperature of 25°C (max 32°C) and an average impedance of 142 Ω (max 171 Ω), leading to definitive termination of AT and restoration of sinus rhythm. After a waiting period of 20 minutes, the tachycardia was no longer observed.

A total of 8 minutes of RF ablation was delivered. The patient tolerated the procedure well, and there were no complications.

During the follow-up, patient remained in sinus rhythm on oral anticoagulation (Apixaban 5 mg twice per day).

DISCUSSION

Recurrent AT can result from the presence of residual atrial arrhythmogenic substrate after AF ablation.[6] The electrophysiological mechanisms underlying most post-AF ablation AT is represented by macro–reentry related to gaps in ablation lines.[6]

Atrial structures such as left atrial PW, IAS, LAA, and thoracic veins such as SVC and CS are major sources of non-PV triggers responsible for atrial tachyarrhythmia recurrence.[8]

Septal ATs can be relatively resistant to catheter ablation and tend to recur during follow-up[6] because of their deep intramural location and the difficulty in achieving good contact and stability of the ablation catheter on the left side of the IAS.[9,10]

In our case the focus of AT appeared to be in the IAS. Both the thickness of the septum and the prolonged ablation required for termination suggested a deep intramural location. The challenge of

A

B

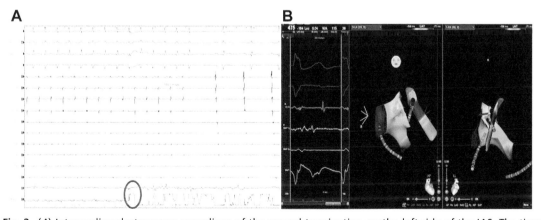

Fig. 2. (A) Intracardiac electrograms recordings of the second termination on the left side of the IAS. The time needed from ablation start to sinus rhythm restoration was 3412 ms. The red circle shows the earliest potential recorded from the ablation catheter and the beginning of ablation.(B) CARTO-3D voltage map showing early potential (−164 ms) and corresponding far-field electrograms on the left side of the IAS before the second termination in anteroposterior and left lateral views.

A

RA   IAS   LA

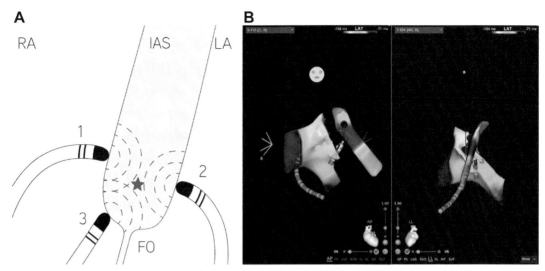

B

Fig. 3. (*A*) Digital drawing showing the first termination point on the right side of the IAS (1), the second termination point on the left side of the IAS (2), the third termination point on the fossa ovalis (3), and a potential intramural position of the AT focus inside the IAS (red star).(*B*) CARTO-3D map showing the 3 points of termination (blue dots) in anteroposterior and left lateral views.

achieving effective ablation using unipolar energy delivery prompted the decision to opt for a bipolar approach.

This method was first used for posteroseptal accessory pathway ablation, when standard unipolar ablation was ineffective, and then it was used for the treatment of VTs originating from the outflow tract, summit, septum, and base of the left ventricle.[11]

With B-RFCA the RF current flows between distal electrodes of 2 separate ablation catheters located on the opposite sides of the target substrate, instead of traveling to an indifferent electrode placed on the patient surface.

B-RFCA was proved to be highly effective at creating larger lesions and at improving the transmurality of lesions,[12,13] thus increasing the chance of success in ablating deep intramural circuits because the inability to create transmural lesions has been shown to be a cause of ablation failure.[14]

The improvement in lesion transmurality can be attributed to several mechanisms, such as thermal synergy between the catheter tips due to

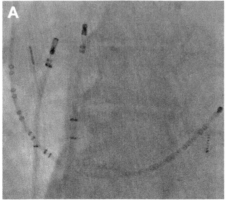

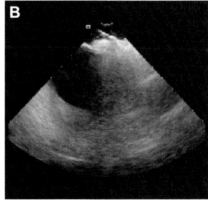

Fig. 4. (*A*) Fluoroscopic anteroposterior image showing the 2 catheters on both sides of the IAS during the bipolar RF energy delivery. An thermocool SF (TSF) catheter is in the left atrium and the other TSF catheter is in the right atrium, together with the ICE probe. (*B*) Intracardiac echocardiographic image showing an TSF catheter in contact with the right side of the IAS and the other TSF catheter at the same level on the other side of the septum. The remarkable thickness of the IAS can be appreciated in this image.

simultaneous heating, higher current density resulting in concentrated thermal injury, and enhanced ablation effectiveness.[12]

In vitro experiments have shown that although sequential unipolar RF could not achieve transmurality in tissue thicker than 15 mm, B-RFCA was able to do so in tissue as deep as 25 mm.[12] These findings are consistent with those of Gizurarson and colleagues, who showed the production of significantly deeper lesions using B-RFCA, without increasing the lesion width, in comparison with standard unipolar ablation.[15]

The effectiveness and safety of B-RFCA are increasingly gaining recognition and despite adding the cost of an additional catheter, the bipolar ablation strategy may result in improved outcomes and shorter procedural times.[13]

A limitation of unipolar ablation is that current flow tends to follow the path of least electrical resistance, potentially deviating from the intended target area. Bipolar ablation overcomes this issue by directing energy through the septum between the 2 catheter tips, ensuring delivery to the desired location.[13]

Limitations in the delivery of RF energy in bipolar fashion include the limited availability of specific devices and the fact that the safety profile of B-RFCA has not been fully determined, yet.

Other authors have pointed out that similar to conventional unipolar ablation, the use of B-RFCA should be assisted with temperature monitoring at the intracardiac return electrode to prevent adverse events related to overheating.[11] Because data on tissue temperature during B-RFCA ablation are limited, monitoring of the return catheter temperature is recommended to avoid core overheating and steam popping.[11]

Another adverse event that should be considered when using B-RFCA is the possibility of an iatrogenic atrial or ventricular septal defect due to the high current density across the septum.

In our case, we used ICE to improve the stability of the catheters and determine their exact position during RF energy delivery, and this can additionally improve outcomes and safety during B-RFCA because options to measure contact force from both catheters during B-RFCA are limited.

SUMMARY

Ablation of atrial tachycardia originating from the septum could be challenging due to a deep intramural location. Our case shows the safety and effectiveness of bipolar radiofrequency ablation to terminate a septal focal AT occurring in a patient with previous AF ablations.

CLINICS CARE POINTS

- Effectiveness for deep locations: B-RFCA can be especially effective for ablation in challenging deep intramural locations, such as the interatrial septum.
- Transmurality: Compared with unipolar ablation, B-RFCA offers an enhanced ability to create transmural lesions, which can be crucial for long-term efficacy.
- Potential for septal defects: High current density across the septum during B-RFCA may introduce a risk for creating iatrogenic septal defects.
- Limited device availability: Not all health-care facilities may have access to the necessary equipment for B-RFCA, potentially limiting its widespread adoption.

DISCLOSURE

Dr Natale is a consultant for Abbott, Baylis, Biosense Webster, Biotronik, Boston Scientific, and Medtronic. All other authors have reported that they have no relationships relevant to the contents of this paper to disclose.

REFERENCES

1. Colilla S, Crow A, Petkun W, et al. Estimates of current and future incidence and prevalence of atrial fibrillation in the U.S. Adult population. Am J Cardiol 2013;112(8):1142–7.
2. Haïssaguerre M, Jaïs P, Shah DC, et al. Spontaneous initiation of atrial fibrillation by ectopic beats originating in the pulmonary veins. N Engl J Med 1998;339(10):659–66.
3. Natale A, Pisano E, Shewchik J, et al. First human experience with pulmonary vein isolation using a through-the-balloon circumferential ultrasound ablation system for recurrent atrial fibrillation. Circulation 2000;102(16):1879–82.
4. Romero J, Gianni C, Natale A, et al. What is the appropriate lesion set for ablation in patients with persistent atrial fibrillation? Curr Treat Options Cardiovasc Med 2017;19(5):35.
5. Della Rocca DG, Di Biase L, Mohanty S, et al. Targeting non-pulmonary vein triggers in persistent atrial fibrillation: results from a prospective, multicentre, observational registry. EP Eur 2021;23(12):1939–49.
6. Chae S, Oral H, Good E, et al. Atrial tachycardia after circumferential pulmonary vein ablation of atrial fibrillation. J Am Coll Cardiol 2007;50(18):1781–7.

7. Hall B, Jeevanantham V, Simon R, et al. Variation in left atrial transmural wall thickness at sites commonly targeted for ablation of atrial fibrillation. J Intervent Card Electrophysiol 2007;17(2):127–32.

8. Della Rocca DG, Tarantino N, Trivedi C, et al. Nonpulmonary vein triggers in nonparoxysmal atrial fibrillation: implications of pathophysiology for catheter ablation. J Cardiovasc Electrophysiol 2020; 31(8):2154–67.

9. Leonelli F, Bagliani G, Boriani G, et al. Arrhythmias originating in the atria. Card Electrophysiol Clin 2017;9(3):383–409.

10. Heck PM, Rosso R, Kistler PM. The challenging face of focal atrial tachycardia in the post AF ablation era. J Cardiovasc Electrophysiol 2011;22(7): 832–8.

11. Futyma P, Ciąpała K, Głuszczyk R, et al. Bipolar ablation of refractory atrial and ventricular arrhythmias: importance of temperature values of intracardiac return electrodes. J Cardiovasc Electrophysiol 2019; 30(9):1718–26.

12. Koruth JS, Dukkipati S, Miller MA, et al. Bipolar irrigated radiofrequency ablation: a therapeutic option for refractory intramural atrial and ventricular tachycardia circuits. Heart Rhythm 2012;9(12):1932–41.

13. Sivagangabalan G, Barry MA, Huang K, et al. Bipolar ablation of the interventricular septum is more efficient at creating a transmural line than sequential unipolar ablation. Pacing Clin Electrophysiol 2010; 33(1):16–26.

14. Melby SJ, Lee AM, Zierer A, et al. Atrial fibrillation propagates through gaps in ablation lines: implications for ablative treatment of atrial fibrillation. Heart Rhythm 2008;5(9):1296–301.

15. Gizurarson S, Spears D, Sivagangabalan G, et al. Bipolar ablation for deep intra-myocardial circuits: human ex vivo development and in vivo experience. Europace 2014;16(11):1684–8.

Catheter Ablation of Idiopathic Epicardial Outflow Tract Premature Ventricular Contractions
A Case Report and Review of the Literature

Jose Aguilera, MD[a], Juan Cabrera, MD[b], Luis Carlos Saenz, MD[b], Pasquale Santangeli, MD, PhD[a],*

KEYWORDS

- Idiopathic ventricular arrhythmias • Ventricular arrhythmia ablation
- Premature ventricular contraction • Epicardial catheter ablation

KEY POINTS

- Most idiopathic ventricular arrhythmias (VAs) originate from perivalvular areas, including the right ventricular or left ventricular outflow tract, periaortic, mitral, and tricuspid annuli, which can be successfully ablated endocardially.
- A small percentage of idiopathic VAs originate from the epicardium, but ablation from adjacent endocardial structures can be attempted. In other cases, ablation through the coronary venous system is possible, including radiofrequency ablation or ethanol injection. It is important to delineate the coronary anatomy before ablating in the coronary venous system.
- Direct epicardial access for ablation of idiopathic VAs has generally low yield due to the risk of injury to coronary arteries and the presence of a thick layer of fat in the usual perivalvular region.
- Epicardial mapping still has a role whenever activation mapping from multiple accessible endocardial or coronary venous/intramural sites yields poor results and no response is observed with ablation from usual anatomic sites.

 Video content accompanies this article at http://www.cardiacep.theclinics.com.

INTRODUCTION

Premature ventricular contractions (PVCs) in the absence of evident structural heart disease are termed idiopathic PVCs. Frequent idiopathic PVCs can be symptomatic, and when the PVC burden is high, it can be associated with the development of left ventricular dysfunction. Catheter ablation of idiopathic PVCs is an effective and safe treatment option but can be challenging. The authors present a case of frequent symptomatic PVCs successfully treated with epicardial catheter ablation.

HISTORY OF PRESENTATION

A 30-year-old woman with a history of frequent symptomatic monomorphic PVCs presents for evaluation after a prior unsuccessful ablation procedure at an outside hospital at the age of 29. As per outside hospital records, her PVC was mapped

[a] Section of Cardiac Pacing and Electrophysiology, Heart and Vascular Institute, Cleveland Clinic, Cleveland, Ohio, USA; [b] Section of Electrophysiology, Fundación Cardioinfantil, Bogotá, Colombia
* Corresponding author. 9500 Euclid Avenue, Cleveland, OH 44195.
E-mail address: santanp3@ccf.org
Twitter: @Dr_Santangeli (P.S.)

Card Electrophysiol Clin 16 (2024) 187–193
https://doi.org/10.1016/j.ccep.2023.10.005
1877-9182/24/© 2023 Elsevier Inc. All rights reserved.

endocardially in the left ventricle (LVOT), right ventricular outflow tract (RVOT), and proximal coronary venous system with a suspicion for left ventricular summit origin, but an optimal ablation site was not identified. She was started on sotalol 160 mg twice a day but continues to have symptoms of palpitations with high PVC burden.

PAST MEDICAL HISTORY

Her other medical problems include obesity (body mass index: 42 kg/m^2).

INVESTIGATIONS

Baseline 12-lead electrocardiogram showed sinus rhythm with narrow QRS and frequent PVCs in a bigeminal pattern (**Fig. 1**). The PVC had a left bundle branch block morphology, a rightward-inferior axis with a precordial R-wave transition at V3 to V4. Lead "I" had a "QS" pattern that suggested possible epicardial origin.[1–4] A 24-hour ambulatory monitoring revealed frequent monomorphic PVCs, greater than 42,000 per 24 hours (36%) without sustained ventricular tachycardia. Cardiac magnetic resonance (CMR) with gadolinium showed mildly reduced left ventricular ejection fraction (LVEF) of 50% with significant dyssynchrony but without evidence of scar or inflammation on late gadolinium enhancement imaging or T2-weighted imaging, respectively (**Fig. 2**).

MANAGEMENT

With a PVC burden above 20% and symptoms, the decision was made to perform a redo PVC ablation. Given previously failed endocardial ablation, concerns that the previous mapping attempt did not include the distal coronary venous system to bracket the earliest activation site, and suspected epicardial origin based on QS pattern in lead I, the authors were prepared to obtain direct epicardial access in case of inadequate mapping/ablation results from accessible endocardial or coronary venous sites.

ABLATION PROCEDURE
Set-Up

The procedure was done under moderate sedation provided by the anesthesia team. Vascular access was obtained with ultrasound guidance of the right femoral vein, left femoral vein, and right femoral artery. The procedure was planned with 3-dimensional mapping system guidance (CARTO, Biosense Webster, Irvine, CA, USA), including a intracardiac echocardiogram using CARTO Sound software (Biosense Webster, Irvine, CA, USA).

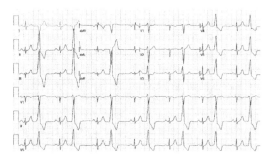

Fig. 1. 12-lead electrocardiogram showing sinus rhythm with narrow QRS and frequent premature ventricular contraction in a bigeminal pattern.

Endocardial Map

An irrigated, contact-force sensing, ablation catheter Thermocool ST-SF (Biosense Webster, Irvine, CA, USA) was used for activation mapping of the PVC. The authors mapped thoroughly in the right and left ventricles with the latter via transseptal approach. The best ablation site was identified to have an electrogram (EGM) occurring 20 minutes pre-QRS but with far-field appearance (**Fig. 3**).

Coronary Venous System Mapping and Ablation

Next, the authors mapped in the coronary venous system. A deflectable Agilis sheath (St. Jude Medical, St. Paul, MN, USA) was placed in the coronary sinus (CS). A contrast injection was done to define anatomy. The great cardiac vein (GCV) and anterior interventricular vein (AIV) had a normal course. The AIV had septal perforator tributaries that were identified in right anterior oblique and left anterior oblique caudal projections (**Fig. 4**A). The GCV, AIV, and septal perforators were mapped with a

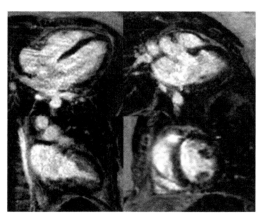

Fig. 2. Cardiac magnetic resonance with late gadolinium enhancement imaging showing no evidence of scar or inflammation.

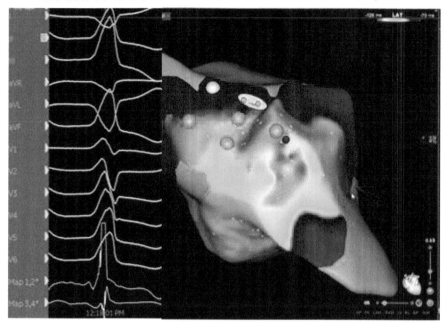

Fig. 3. (A) Electrogram of the earliest activation site in the left ventricular endocardium, pre-QRS ∼20 minutes but far-field appearance in the distal bipole of the ablation catheter (Map 1, 2). (B) Activation of the endocardial points, showing the earliest site in the anterior midleft ventricle.

2-French decapolar catheter (EPStar, Baylis, Toronto, Ontario, Canada) (Fig. 4B). The earliest activation site in the coronary venous system was in the mid-AIV, distal from the atrio-ventricular groove. Activation was later in the septal perforator branches compared with the mid-AIV, suggesting that the PVC origin was unlikely to be intramural. Fig. 5.

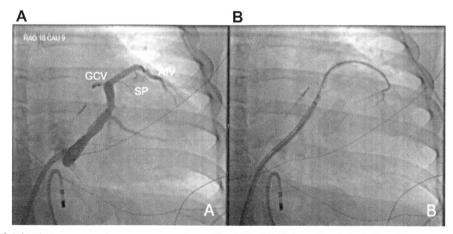

Fig. 4. (A) Selective coronary sinus venogram shows the AIV with SP branches tributaries, this was confirmed to be SP on different fluoroscopy projection. (B) A 2-French decapolar EP star catheter in a septal perforator branch adjacent to the earliest breakout site in the mid-AIV to map the PVC activation. AIV, anterior interventricular vein; GCV, great cardiac vein; PVC, premature ventricular contraction; SP,septal perforator.

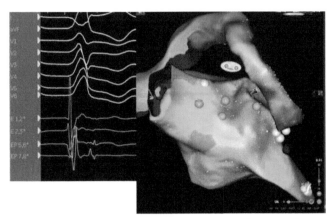

Septal Perforator

Mid-AIV

Fig. 5. Activation mapping with a decapolar catheter in the mid-AIV and septal perforators. The earliest activation site in the coronary venous system is in the mid-AIV. AIV, anterior interventricular vein.

The ablation catheter was then advanced into the AIV, at the site of earliest activation. Here the local EGM was 24 minutes pre-QRS and pacing showed a good pace match (95%) (**Fig. 6**). Before ablation, a coronary angiogram was obtained in different projections to evaluate proximity to the coronary arteries. The authors delineated a distance of at least 0.6 cm from the tip of the ablation catheter to the midleft anterior descending artery which was felt to be safe. Radiofrequency ablation (RFA) was delivered in the mid-AIV starting on 20 W of power and with careful attention to impedance changes. Ablation here did not have any effect on the PVCs. Next, the authors delivered RFA at anatomically adjacent vantage points in the midseptal LVOT and RVOT, opposite to the site of earliest activation

in the AIV, but this did not influence PVC frequency either (**Fig. 7**).

Epicardial Mapping and Ablation

Given the lack of adequate ablation targets and ablation effect from multiple accessible LVOT and RVOT sites as well from within the CS, the authors decided to map the epicardium. Subxiphoid percutaneous epicardial access was obtained and activation mapping of the epicardium was performed. The earliest activation site was found to be in the midleft ventricle at the site opposite of the earliest endocardial activation within the left ventricle (**Fig. 8** and Video 1). Here the local bipolar EGM was 43 minutes pre-QRS of the PVC (**Fig. 9**). Given these characteristic features of an optimal ablation site, the authors delivered RFA (40–50W for

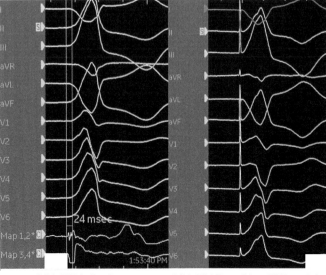

Mid-AIV Activation   Mid-AIV Pace Map 95% match

Fig. 6. Ablation catheter placed in the mid-AIV at the site of earliest activation. Here the distal bipole is pre-QRS 24 milliseconds. Pace match is good 95%. AIV, anterior interventricular vein.

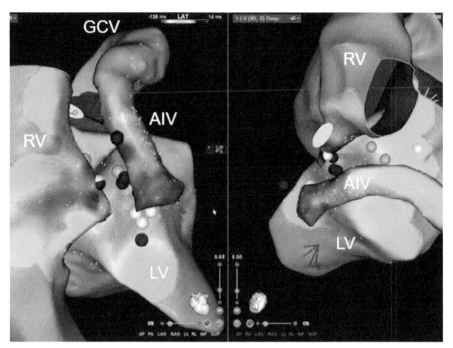

Fig. 7. Activation map of the PVC in the right ventricle, left ventricle, and coronary venous system with the ablation lesions (*red dots*) in the mid-AIV and midleft ventricle. No changes in PVC frequency was seen after those ablations. AIV, anterior interventricular vein; GCV,great cardiac vein; LV, left ventricle; PVC, premature ventricular contraction; RV,right ventricle.

180 seconds) after coronary angiogram showed safe coronary distance (**Fig. 10**).

After a few seconds, the PVC frequency decreased and subsequently disappeared completely (Video 2). A repeat coronary angiogram was completed postablation, confirming no injury to the coronary arteries.

Case Conclusion

After 45 minutes of monitoring, the patient remained in normal sinus rhythm without PVCs. She tolerated

the procedure with no complications. She was discharged home the following day off sotalol. On 1-month follow-up, the 15-day cardiac monitor showed less than 0.1% PVC burden and repeated CMR showed improvement of LVEF from 50% to 60%.

DISCUSSION

Most idiopathic ventricular arrhythmias (VAs) originate from the perivalvular anatomic regions,

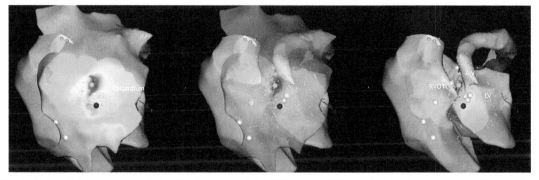

Fig. 8. Epicardial and endocardial activation map of the PVC with 3 different levels of transparency of the epicardial map, showing earliest focal site of activation in the epicardium (*green dot*) and the relation with the left ventricle and mid-AIV. AIV, anterior interventricular vein; LV,left ventricle; PVC, premature ventricular contraction; RVOT, right ventricular outflow tract.

A   B   C

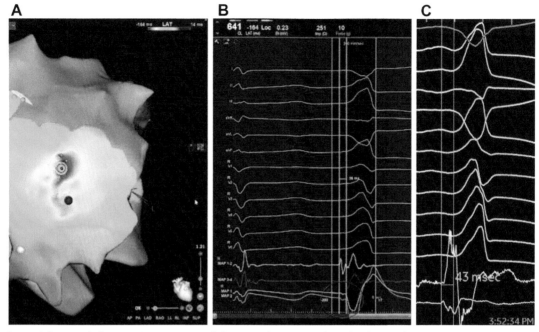

Fig. 9. (*A*) Epicardial activation mapping of the PVC, showing earliest focal site of activation (*green dot*). The phrenic nerve was located (*white dot*) (*B*) At the earliest site, unipolar electrogram shows "QS pattern." (*C*) Bipolar electrogram showed pre-QRS 43 milliseconds at site of earliest activation. PVC, premature ventricular contraction.

including the RVOT, LVOT, aortic valve, sinus of Valsalva, pulmonic valve, and mitral and tricuspid annuli.[5] Other less frequent locations include the papillary muscle, left fascicular conduction system, and left ventricular myocardium. This case is unique in that the PVC site of origin was epicardial in the midleft anterior ventricle, significantly distant from the typical perivalvular area.

For perivalvular epicardial PVCs, mapping is usually performed from the coronary venous system but in one-third of cases, ablation is precluded due to proximity to the coronary arteries or inability

to advance the ablation catheter into the coronary venous branches.[1-3] Occasionally, the VA origin is intramural, and ethanol ablation delivered retrograde via the coronary venous system is a viable treatment option.[6,7] In the authors' case, activation mapping inside the venous septal perforator branches was found to be later compared with the mid AIV, suggesting that the origin was not intramural (See **Fig. 5**).

Direct epicardial puncture for mapping and ablation of idiopathic VAs, has typically been considered of low yield due to the presence of

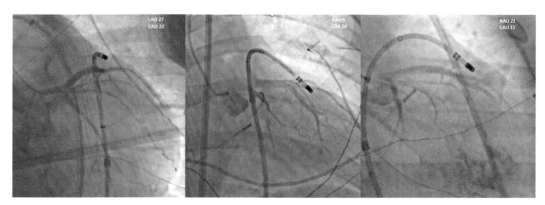

Fig. 10. Selective coronary angiogram in different projections of the left main coronary artery with the ablation catheter located in the epicardium, at the site of earliest activation site of the PVC. PVC, premature ventricular contraction

major epicardial vessels at the common perivalvular locations. Additionally, the presence of a thick layer of epicardial fat around this area can result in ineffective ablation lesions.[3,8]

The authors' case was unique in the fact that the epicardial site of origin was in the para-septal mid-left ventricle, far from the major proximal coronary arteries and from the region of epicardial fat which is most represented in the basal perivalvular region.

DISCLOSURE

J. Aguilera: Nothing to disclose. Pasquale Santangeli: Consultant for Biosense Webster, Abbott, Boston Scientific and Medtronic. J. Cabrera: Nothing to disclose. L. C. Saenz: Consultant for Biosense Webster, Abbott.

SUPPLEMENTARY DATA

Supplementary data related to this article can be found online at https://doi.org/10.1016/j.ccep.2023.10.005.

REFERENCES

1. Frankel DS, Mountantonakis SE, Dahu MI, et al. Elimination of ventricular arrhythmias originating from the anterior interventricular vein with ablation in the right ventricular outflow tract. Circulation Arrhythmia and electrophysiology 2014;7:984–5.

2. Jauregui Abularach ME, Campos B, Park KM, et al. Ablation of ventricular arrhythmias arising near the anterior epicardial veins from the left sinus of Valsalva region: ECG features, anatomic distance, and outcome. Heart Rhythm 2012;9:865–73.

3. Santangeli P, Marchlinski FE, Zado ES, et al. Percutaneous epicardial ablation of ventricular arrhythmias arising from the left ventricular summit: outcomes and ECG correlates of success. Circulation Arrhythmia and electrophysiology 2015. https://doi.org/10.1161/CIRCEP.114.002377.

4. Valles E, Bazan V, Marchlinski FE. ECG criteria to identify epicardial ventricular tachycardia in nonischemic cardiomyopathy. Circulation Arrhythmia and electrophysiology 2010;3:63–71.

5. Enriquez A, Baranchuk A, Briceno D, et al. How to use the 12-lead ECG to predict the site of origin of idiopathic ventricular arrhythmias. Heart Rhythm 2019;16:1538–44.

6. Fuentes Rojas SC, Malahfji M, Tavares L, et al. Acute and long-term scar characterization of venous ethanol ablation in the left ventricular summit. JACC Clin Electrophysiol 2023;9:28–39.

7. Neira V, Santangeli P, Futyma P, et al. Ablation strategies for intramural ventricular arrhythmias. Heart Rhythm 2020;17:1176–84.

8. Yamada T, McElderry HT, Doppalapudi H, et al. Idiopathic ventricular arrhythmias originating from the left ventricular summit: anatomic concepts relevant to ablation. Circulation Arrhythmia and electrophysiology 2010;3:616–23.

Pediatric and Familial Genetic Arrhythmia Syndromes–Evaluation of Prolonged QTc–Differential Diagnosis and what You Need to Know

Mary C. Niu, MD[a], Susan P. Etheridge, MD[a], Martin Tristani-Firouzi, MD[a],
Christina Y. Miyake, MD, MS[b],*

KEYWORDS

- Prolonged QT • QTc • Long QT syndrome • Timothy syndrome • CALM • Calmodulinopathy
- TANGO2 • Andersen-Tawil syndrome

KEY POINTS

- The most common genetic cause of QTc prolongation is long QT syndrome types 1, 2, and 3.
- There are also other less common syndromes associated with QTc prolongation that are crucial to recognize because of their significant association with a high risk of lethal arrhythmias and sudden death.
- Recognizing signs and symptoms of each particular disease is important to making the correct diagnosis.

INTRODUCTION

The following case series comprises 4 different cases of QTc prolongation and highlights the key features of each case while offering a practical approach to diagnosing and managing these patients. Common and rare genetic conditions associated with prolonged QTc are presented. For each case, review the history, electrocardiograms (ECGs), and rhythm tracings. Carefully consider the differential diagnosis and treatment strategy before delving into the discussion and learning about each case.

CASE 1
Clinical Presentation

A 5-year-old girl presents to clinic for multiple episodes of syncope. One event occurred during a school fire alarm. She denies any prodromal symptoms. Her ECG (**Fig. 1**) demonstrates sinus bradycardia and significant QTc prolongation of 510 milliseconds; the T waves are notched and bifid. Her family history is notable for her mother dying suddenly. Her mother was found deceased next to her bed in the early morning when this patient was 3 months old.

Funding: C.Y. Miyake is funded through NHLBI, United States K23HL136932.
[a] Department of Pediatric Cardiology, University of Utah and Primary Children's Hospital, 100 Mario Capecchi Drive, Salt Lake City, UT 84113, USA; [b] Department of Pediatrics, Division of Cardiology, Texas Children's Hospital and Baylor College of Medicine, 6651 Main Street, Houston, TX 77003, USA
* Corresponding author.
E-mail address: cymiyake@bcm.edu

Card Electrophysiol Clin 16 (2024) 195–202
https://doi.org/10.1016/j.ccep.2023.10.006

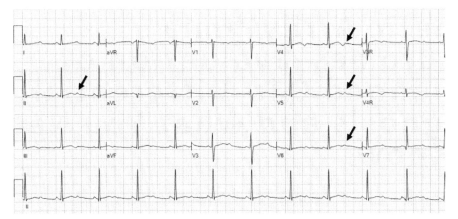

Fig. 1. ECG demonstrates a QTc of 510 milliseconds. The arrows point out prominent U waves and bifid T waves.

Discussion

This case underscores the critical role of patient and family history in diagnosing long QT syndrome (LQTS). The red flag signs and symptoms from this family's history include

1. This child is far younger than typical for vasovagal syncope and has no prodromal symptoms.
2. Syncope was triggered by loud noises, a known trigger for long QT type 2.
3. Her mother died suddenly 3 months postpartum after the birth of this child and was found in the early morning next to her bed. Postpartum and death in early morning hours due to alarm clocks are classic triggers for arrhythmias and sudden death in long QT type 2.

In a patient with syncope, triggers like exertion, startle, surprise, or emotional stress are red flags for an arrhythmogenic cardiac events. In such cases, an ECG is mandatory, and for this patient, makes the diagnosis of LQTS. When the QTc is borderline, provocative testing such as an exercise treadmill can be used to assess for abnormal QTc prolongation (at peak exercise in LQT1 and during recovery in LQT2). Treadmill testing is not helpful in LQT3 or other LQT-related syndromes. The ECG for the patient shows classic T wave changes in LQT2: notched and bifid T waves. Genetic testing is indicated, because identifying the affected gene and gene variant carries significant implications for prognosis and therapy. Cascade screening of all first-degree relatives is crucial to identify at-risk individuals. Interpreting genetic results can be complex, and the process of deciding which relatives should undergo screening is not always straightforward. Therefore, it is advisable to have genetic testing conducted at a facility with access to genetic counselors who can offer expert guidance in these matters. In this patient's case, a mutation in the pore region of KCNH2 was detected; pore region mutations are associated with a higher symptom burden and an increased risk for arrhythmia-related cardiac events.[1]

There are several different genetic disorders that cause QTc prolongation, but by far, the most common genetic cause is LQTS types 1, 2 and 3. Some rarer syndromes such as Timothy syndrome and calmodulinopathies are associated with the most severe disease forms. Most LQTS is inherited in an autosomal-dominant manner. LQT1 and LQT2 are caused by loss-of-function variants in the KCNQ1 and KCNH2 potassium channels, respectively. LQT1 is characterized by cardiac events during adrenaline surges, particularly sports, with swimming being a specific trigger. Triggers for LQT2 are startle, loud noises, and emotion (eg, fear or anxiety). Importantly, women with LQT2 have a reduced risk for cardiac events during pregnancy but an increased risk during the 9-month postpartum period,[2] as illustrated by this patient's mother. Less common than types 1 and 2, LQT3 is caused by a gain-of-function in the sodium channel SCN5A, and cardiac events typically occur during times of bradycardia such as sleep.

Treatment of LQTS includes medical therapy and life-style counseling to avoid disease-specific triggers. Nonselective beta blockers, such as nadolol and propranolol, are the mainstay of therapy[3,4] for patients who are both genotype and phenotype positive. In LQT3, mexiletine can reduce the occurrence of arrhythmic events by reducing the QT interval.[5] Adjunctive therapies, including left cardiac sympathetic denervation, can be added to tailor the management strategy to the patient's disease, and implantable cardioverter defibrillators are implanted if symptoms persist despite therapy. Gene therapy may be an option in the future.

CASES 2 AND 3
Clinical Presentation

Two unrelated full-term newborn infants with brady-cardia to the 60s are brought to the intensive care unit (ICU). ECGs on both infants reveal ventricular septal defects. The ECGs of both babies are shown in **Fig. 2**. Baby A has a QTc of 690 milliseconds with T wave alternans and is a normal-appearing infant. Baby B has a QTc of 655 milliseconds, has a round facies with 4,5 syndactyly of the left hand and bilateral 2,3 toe syndactyly. Neither infant has any concerning family history.

Both ECGs demonstrate profound QTc prolongation resulting in functional 2:1 atrioventricular (AV) block. Genetic testing is performed. Baby A has no known LQTS-associated variants. Baby B is found to have a de novo pathogenic variant in CACNA1C.

Discussion

Both cases represent severe infantile presentations of long QT syndrome associated with a high risk for life-threatening arrhythmias and sudden cardiac death (SCD). When the QTc interval is markedly prolonged, the heart rate is slow because of functional block. This means that the ventricle is still refractory because of prolonged repolarization such that the next sinus *P* wave cannot conduct, resulting in 2:1 conduction where every other *P* wave results in ventricular contraction. This finding does not signify disease within the conduction system but rather, severe prolongation in ventricular repolarization. T-wave alternans (TWA) is an important phenomenon to recognize and can be seen when there is marked QTc prolongation. TWA is characterized by beat-to-beat fluctuations in the shape or amplitude of the T wave. A sign of repolarization instability, TWA is associated with ventricular arrhythmias and increased risk of sudden cardiac arrest.[6]

LQTS should be considered in the differential diagnosis for fetal or neonatal AV block as well as fetal bradycardia. In the absence of symptoms or arrhythmias, these features still warrant investigation and treatment, even when genetic testing is negative. Genetic factors are estimated to account for 75% to 80% of LQTS cases. As such, it is imperative that test results be interpreted within the clinical context.[7] A negative genetic test does not exclude disease, particularly when the QTc is markedly prolonged and there is a strong clinical suspicion for LQTS. Moreover, a negative test alone should not dictate treatment. Rather, the clinical context should drive treatment and guide the diagnostic process.

In severe cases of QTc prolongation, it is important to consider rare diseases. Despite negative commercial gene testing, Baby A was monitored in the hospital for 1 month, during which time propranolol treatment was initiated and a single

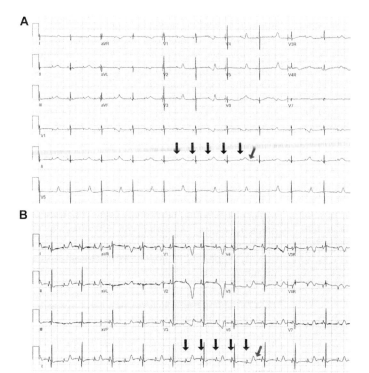

Fig. 2. (*A*) ECG for Baby A who has no dysmorphic features. The QTc is 690 milliseconds. (*B*) ECG for Baby B, who has a round facies, syndactyly, and clinodactyly. The QTc is 655 milliseconds. For both ECGs, black arrows indicate *P* waves; red arrows mark the end of the T wave.

chamber pacemaker implanted. During this time, extended sequencing was performed and identified a de novo variant in *CALM3* that was not present on commercial genetic testing at that time. This patient was the first *CALM3* patient identified, but subsequent *CALM3* patients have been identified.[8] *CALM* mutations are now a standard part of most commercial LQTS gene testing panels.

Baby A was diagnosed with CALM3-related calmodulinopathy. Calmodulinopathies are caused by pathogenic heterozygous variants in any of the 3 genes (*CALM 1–3*) that encode identical calmodulin (CaM) Ca^{2+} signaling proteins.[9] Patients express a varied severe phenotype of LQTS, catecholaminergic polymorphic ventricular tachycardia, sudden explained death, idiopathic ventricular fibrillation, hypertrophic cardiomyopathy, or mixed disease. The mean QTc duration from CALM-LQTS probands in the 2023 registry was 579 plus or minus 78 milliseconds,[7,8] and over half of the 2019 registry patients experienced recurrent cardiac events despite management strategies that included combination therapy with beta blockers, sodium channel blockers, other antiarrhythmics, sympathetic denervation, and pacing.[7,8]

Baby B was diagnosed with Timothy syndrome (TS), a rare, autosomal-dominant multisystem disorder caused by pathogenic variants in the *CACNA1C* gene that encodes the L-type calcium channel, Cav1.2. TS is characterized by a constellation of neurodevelopmental, facial, hand/foot, and cardiac features. Individuals with TS demonstrate global developmental delays and may also be diagnosed with autism spectrum disorders. Facial features include round facies, a flat nasal bridge, low-set ears, and thin upper lip. Additional extracardiac manifestations include unilateral or bilateral cutaneous syndactyl.[10] (**Fig. 3**)

The cardiac phenotype of TS includes congenital heart defects and marked QTc prolongation, typically more than 500 milliseconds, that predisposes the patient to malignant arrhythmias and SCD. For this reason, it is imperative to initiate treatment. Management is aimed at stabilizing repolarization, reducing the frequency and propensity for ventricular arrhythmias, and providing rescue therapy for malignant arrhythmias. A combination of interventions, including medications, rate stabilization through pacing, implantation of an implantable cardioverter-defibrillator (ICD), and LCSD are frequently required. Baby B had a pacemaker placed the first week of life, before diagnostic genetic testing results were available. Because of persistent TWA despite propranolol and mexiletine, an epicardial ICD was placed and an LCSD performed concurrently. He has received appropriate ICD discharges but is doing well as a teenager.

CASE 4
Clinical Presentation

A 5-year-old boy presents to the emergency room with a 3-day history of viral symptoms, poor oral intake, lethargy, and slurred speech. His parents report he has been walking like a "drunk sailor" and falling. His past medical history is notable for delayed developmental milestones, episodic ataxia, and dysarthria. Laboratory values are significant for hypoglycemia and elevated creatinine kinase (CK), alanine transaminase (ALT), and aspartate transaminase (AST). His electrolytes are normal. His ECG demonstrates a QTc of 585 milliseconds and type I Brugada pattern (**Fig. 4**). He has mild systolic dysfunction on echocardiogram. He develops hemodynamically significant torsade de pointes (TdP) in the setting of sinus tachycardia. Despite intravenous magnesium, esmolol, lidocaine, and defibrillation, TdP is recalcitrant. He is placed onto extracorporeal membrane oxygenation.

Discussion

This patient has clinical features classic for TANGO2 deficiency disorder (TDD), a rare disease caused by biallelic variants in the *TANGO2* gene.[11] Affected children and adults exhibit baseline developmental and cognitive delays, along with dysarthria. Many also have hypothyroidism and seizures. When healthy, the QTc interval is normal. Periods of illness or inadequate oral intake, however, lead to metabolic crisis, defined by the presence of rhabdomyolysis (elevated CK) and prolonged QTc intervals. During crisis, patients can develop life-threatening TdP and systolic dysfunction. Mortality from arrhythmias and cardiac arrest is extremely high.[12] This is an important disease to recognize, because TdP does not respond to conventional long QT treatments. Amiodarone and lidocaine should be avoided. Although there is no specific therapy that suppresses all ventricular tachycardia (VT) episodes, 2 of the most effective options for temporary VT suppression include isoproterenol and atrial pacing above the sinus rate.[12] Nutrition and administration of B vitamins are the sole measures for crisis resolution, including normalization of QTc and cardiac function. B vitamins should be administered as part of routine daily treatment to avoid metabolic crisis.[11,13]

DISCUSSION AND SUMMARY OF 4 CASES: EVALUATING PROLONGED QTc

The cardiologist assessing a patient with QT prolongation is tasked with the following objectives. First, does the patient have genetic LQTS? LQTS

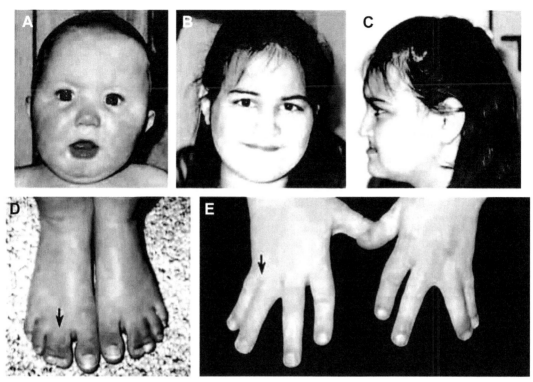

Fig. 3. Clinical manifestations of TS include round face, flat nasal bridge, receding upper jaw, thin upper lip (A–C) and the *arrows* demonstrate syndactyly of the toes (*D*) andn fingers (*E*). (Igor Splawski et al., CaV1.2 Calcium Channel Dysfunction Causes a Multisystem Disorder Including Arrhythmia and Autism, Cell, 119 (1), 2004, 19-31, https://doi.org/10.1016/j.cell.2004.09.011.)

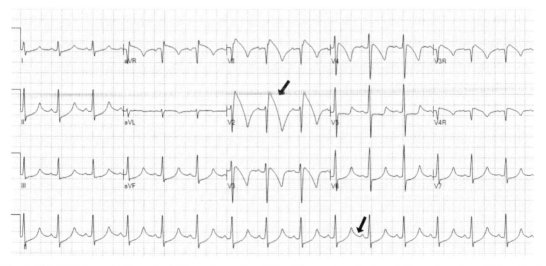

Fig. 4. This ECG shows both marked QTc prolongation, 585 milliseconds and a type 1 Brugada pattern. This patient has neurodevelopmental delays, ataxia, slurred speech and rhabdomyolysis. The top *black arrow* shows the type 1 Brugada pattern. The *bottom arrow* shows marked QTc prolongation. (Miyake CY, Lay EJ, Beach CM, et al. Cardiac crises: Cardiac arrhythmias and cardiomyopathy during TANGO2 deficiency related metabolic crises, Heart Rhythm, 19 (10), 2022, 1673-1681, https://doi.org/10.1016/j.hrthm.2022.05.009.)

affects 1 in 2000 individuals. In the absence of iatrogenic or predisposing factors (eg, QT-prolonging medications, electrolyte abnormalities, thyroid disease, or heart failure),[14] genetic LQTS is the most likely cause of QTc prolongation.

Next, what are the signs and symptoms from the individual's and extended family's history heralding inherited LQTS, and does the collective symptomatology align with a specific LQTS subtype? It is incumbent upon the physician to gather details essential for understanding life-threatening event-triggering circumstances including syncope, seizures, and cardiac arrest. Not only do these triggers help direct the diagnosis toward specific LQTS subtypes, trigger avoidance and management become pivotal to mitigating the risk of future SCD. Although one cannot rely solely on these factors, knowing which triggers are associated with each LQTS subtype and reviewing the T-wave morphology can help clinicians make the diagnosis even before genetic testing returns.

Rare syndromes associated with prolonged QT can be diagnosed through careful physical examination. Familiarity with specific dysmorphisms and extracardiac manifestations can assist in reaching the correct diagnosis. For example, both TS and Andersen-Tawil Syndrome (ATS) are associated with prolonged QTc. A case of ATS is described in the article by Miyake in this issue. The QTc is typically markedly long in TS, whereas in ATS, the length of the QTc varies depending on the presence of U waves, which may not always be seen. Although syndactyl is a shared feature between TS and ATS, the facial dysmorphisms associated with each condition are distinct. Although TDD patients are not dysmorphic, their history of developmental delays, ataxia or balance problems, and dysarthria can pinpoint the diagnosis.

ECG data can also be helpful (**Fig. 5**). LQTS1 patients tend to have early onset, broad-based T waves; LQTS2 patients often have bifid, or notched T waves; and LQTS3 patients can have

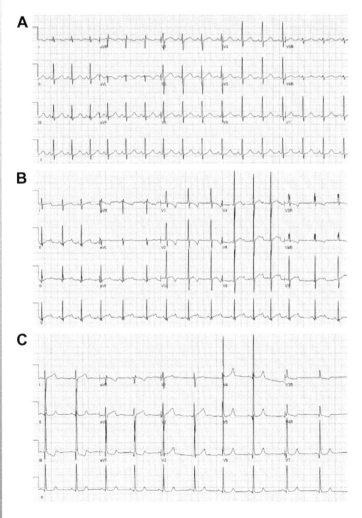

A

B

C

Fig. 5. T-wave morphology can be helpful but is not diagnostic. T waves are broad based in LQT1 (*A*); bifid with prominent U waves in LQT2 (*B*); and have a long isoelectric time before the T-wave in LQT3 (*C*).

Table 1
Description of features among syndromes associated with prolonged QTc

Syndrome	Channel/Protein Effect	Triggers	ECG	Other
LQTS type 1	K (KCNQ1) LOF	Exercise swimming		
LQTS type 1	K (KCNQ1) LOF	Startle, loud noise, emotion, postpartum		
LQTS type 1	NA (SCN5A) GOF	Sleep		
Timothy syndrome	Ca (CACNA1C) GOF		Marked QTc prolongation	Round facies, thin upper lip, low set ears, flat nasal bridge, neurodevelopmental delays, syndactyly
Calmodulinopathy	Ca sensing/ signaling (CALM1, CALM2, CALM3)		Marked QTc prolongation	Mixed phenotype: LQTS, CPVT, cardiomyopathy
Andersen-Tawil syndrome	K (KCNJ2) LOF			Broad forehead, low set ears, small jaw/dental crowding, clinodactyly, 2–3 toe syndactyly
TANGO2 deficiency disorder	Unknown effect (TANGO2)	Fever, illness, not eating	QTc prolongation only when in crisis, type1 Brugada pattern	Neurodevelopmental delays, speech problems (dysarthria), gait abnormalities, rhabdomyolysis when in crisis

long isoelectric ST segments with late-appearing normal morphology T waves.[15] Patients with CALM mutations and TS commonly have profoundly prolonged QT intervals greater than 500 milliseconds, which in the fetus and neonate, can cause bradycardia because of functional 2:1 AV block; TWA may also be present. The presence of QTc prolongation in the setting of rhabdomyolysis in a patient with developmental delays and speech and gait abnormalities can identify TANGO2 deficiency disorder.

Prolonged QTc is a clinical manifestation of several different syndromes, including LQTS, TS, calmodulinopathies, ATS and TANGO2 deficiency disorder, and others. This article provides helpful tips for recognizing different causes of prolonged QTc and associated syndromes (**Table 1**).

CLINICS CARE POINTS

- First line treatment for patients diagnosed with Long QT syndrome is a non-selective beta blocker.

- Prolonged QTc in the presence of syndromic characteristics should raise suspicion for Timothy Syndrome and Anderson-Tawil Syndrome.
- Patients wtih intermittent QTc prolongation in the setting of rhabdomyolysis in a child are at significant risk and should be evaluated for TANGO2 Deficiency Disorder.

DISCLOSURE

M.C. Niu: none; C.Y. Miyake: none.

REFERENCES

1. Moss AJ, Zareba W, Kaufman ES, et al. Increased risk of arrhythmic events in long-QT syndrome with mutations in the pore region of the human ether-a-go-go-related gene potassium channel. Circulation 2002;105(7):794–9.

2. Seth R, Moss AJ, McNitt S, et al. Long QT syndrome and pregnancy. J Am Coll Cardiol 2007;49(10):1092–8.

3. Chockalingam P, Crotti L, Girardengo G, et al. Not all beta-blockers are equal in the management of long QT syndrome types 1 and 2: higher recurrence of events under metoprolol. J Am Coll Cardiol 2012; 60(20):2092–9.

4. Went TR, Sultan W, Sapkota A, et al. A systematic review on the role of betaeta-blockers in reducing cardiac arrhythmias in long QT syndrome subtypes 1-3. Cureus 2021;13(9):e17632.

5. Mazzanti A, Maragna R, Faragli A, et al. Gene-specific therapy with mexiletine reduces arrhythmic events in patients with long QT syndrome type 3. J Am Coll Cardiol 2016;67(9):1053–8.

6. You T, Luo C, Zhang K, et al. Electrophysiological mechanisms underlying T-wave alternans and their role in arrhythmogenesis. Front Physiol 2021;12:614946.

7. Crotti L, Spazzolini C, Tester DJ, et al. Calmodulin mutations and life-threatening cardiac arrhythmias: insights from the International Calmodulinopathy Registry. Eur Heart J 2019;40(35):2964–75.

8. Crotti L, Spazzolini C, Nyegaard M, et al. Clinical presentation of calmodulin mutations: the international calmodulinopathy Registry. Eur Heart J 2023; 44(35):3357–70.

9. Reed GJ, Boczek NJ, Etheridge SP, et al. CALM3 mutation associated with long QT syndrome. Heart Rhythm 2015;12(2):419–22.

10. Napolitano C, Antzelevitch C. Phenotypical manifestations of mutations in the genes encoding subunits of the cardiac voltage-dependent L-type calcium channel. Circ Res 2011;108(5):607–18.

11. Miyake CY, Lay EJ, Soler-Alfonso C, et al. Natural history of TANGO2 deficiency disorder: baseline assessment of 73 patients. Genet Med 2022. https://doi.org/10.1016/j.gim.2022.11.020.

12. Miyake CY, Lay EJ, Beach CM, et al. Cardiac crises: cardiac arrhythmias and cardiomyopathy during TANGO2 deficiency related metabolic crises. Heart Rhythm 2022. https://doi.org/10.1016/j.hrthm.2022.05.009.

13. Sandkuhler SE, Zhang L, Meisner JK, et al. B-complex vitamins for patients with TANGO2-deficiency disorder. J Inherit Metab Dis 2023;46(2):161–2.

14. Kallergis EM, Goudis CA, Simantirakis EN, et al. Mechanisms, risk factors, and management of acquired long QT syndrome: a comprehensive review. Sci World J 2012;2012:212178.

15. Porta-Sanchez A, Spillane DR, Harris L, et al. T-wave morphology analysis in congenital long QT syndrome discriminates patients from healthy individuals. JACC Clin Electrophysiol 2017;3(4):374–81.

Pediatric and Familial Genetic Arrhythmia Syndromes: Evaluation of Bidirectional Ventricular Tachycardia—Differential Diagnosis

Mohammad A. Ebrahim, MD[a], Tam Dan Pham, MD[b], Mary C. Niu, MD[c], Susan P. Etheridge, MD[c], Martin Tristani-Firouzi, MD[c], Christina Y. Miyake, MD, MS[b],*

KEYWORDS

- Bidirectional • Ventricular tachycardia • CPVT • Anderson-Tawil syndrome • TECRL

KEY POINTS

- Bidirectional ventricular tachycardia (VT) is a unique, relatively uncommon condition with a short differential.
- Bidirectional VT is associated with several life-threatening conditions, and physicians must make an accurate diagnosis to guide appropriate management.
- Recognizing the signs and symptoms specific to each disease is essential for arriving at the correct diagnosis.

INTRODUCTION

The following report presents 3 different pediatric and familial cases, with a focus on salient features and practical aspects related to the diagnosis and management of patients with bidirectional ventricular tachycardia (VT). Common and rare genetic conditions associated with bidirectional VT will be presented. For each case, we suggest reading the history, reviewing any electrocardiograms (ECGs) or tracings, and considering your initial differential diagnosis and treatment strategy before proceeding to the discussion and learning about each case.

CASE 1: CLINICAL PRESENTATION

A 15-year-old otherwise healthy boy has a history of recurrent syncope, which began at age 11 years. The first episode occurred during an argument with his father. He regained consciousness after receiving brief cardiopulmonary resuscitation (CPR) from his family. Two subsequent episodes, one while jumping on a trampoline and another while giving a speech in front of his class, resulted in loss of consciousness with seizure-like activity. He quickly returns to his usual self after these events with no postictal confusion or tiredness. He was referred to neurology and cardiology for

[a] Department of Pediatrics, Chest Diseases Hospital, Kuwait University, Jabriya, Block 4, Street 102, Kuwait City, 46300, Kuwait; [b] Department of Pediatrics, Texas Children's Hospital, 6651 Main Street, Houston, TX 77003, USA; [c] Department of Pediatrics, Division of Cardiology, University of Utah and Primary Children's Hospital, 100 Mario Capecchi Drive, Salt Lake City, UT 84113, USA
* Corresponding author.
E-mail address: cymiyake@bcm.edu

Card Electrophysiol Clin 16 (2024) 203–210
https://doi.org/10.1016/j.ccep.2023.10.002
1877-9182/24/© 2023 Elsevier Inc. All rights reserved.

evaluation and his physical examination, ECG, echocardiogram, Holter, electroencephalogram, and head computed tomography were all normal. His family history was unremarkable. A few months later, he was performing at his first dance recital and collapsed while on stage. Bystander CPR was initiated, and a defibrillator successfully converted him back to sinus rhythm. After making a full recovery, he underwent exercise stress testing (EST), which elicited the rhythm shown in **Fig. 1**.

CASE 1: CLINICAL QUESTIONS

1. What is your differential diagnosis for this patient's recurrent syncope and cardiac arrest?
2. What aspects of his history help make the diagnosis?
3. What is the treatment of this patient?

CASE 1: DISCUSSION

This case highlights the importance of recognizing the differential diagnosis for exertional and emotional syncope, which includes both long QT syndrome and catecholaminergic polymorphic ventricular tachycardia (CPVT). This patient's history of syncope triggered by adrenergic stimulation (anger, exertion, anxiety, and fear) with a normal ECG is consistent with CPVT. The patient's sense of normalcy, coupled with the absence of a postictal state after "seizure-like" activity is vital for distinguishing an arrhythmic etiology from a seizure. This is important because patients with heritable arrhythmia syndromes can be misdiagnosed with seizure disorder. Other typical features of CPVT include a structurally normal heart and a normal resting ECG although sinus bradycardia is almost uniformly present. In most cases, the ambulatory Holter monitor is also normal unless the patient happens to have an adrenergic stimulating event while wearing the monitor. If the Holter monitor demonstrates premature ventricular contractions (PVC) or VT, the ectopy tends to cluster only at fastest heart rates. Holter monitors with significant ventricular ectopy burden throughout the day and during sleep are not consistent with CPVT. The gold standard for CPVT diagnosis is an exercise stress test. A modified protocol, which allows the patient to achieve peak heart rates quickly should be considered and can be more useful than following the standard Bruce protocol. This is because some children tire before reaching peak exercise using the Bruce protocol, limiting the ability to trigger VTs. Exercise stress tests typically begin with normal sinus rhythm followed by isolated PVCs that progress to a bigeminal pattern followed by bidirectional or polymorphic VT. Atrial tachycardia (AT) may also occur.[1] The finding of simultaneous VT and AT on EST is not common

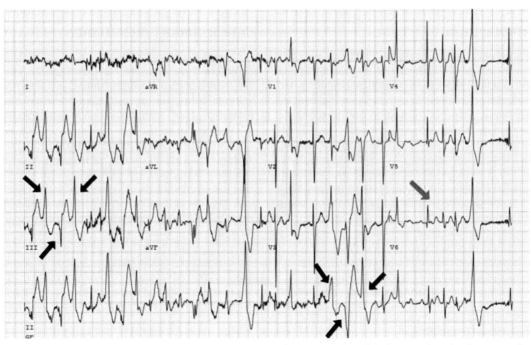

Fig. 1. Case 1 EST. During exercise treadmill testing, there is bidirectional VT (*black arrows*) and a short run of AT (*red arrow*).

in other disorders and helps clinch the diagnosis of CPVT. Genetic testing in this patient revealed a de novo heterozygous variant in the *RYR2* gene, leading to a gain of function in the cardiac Ryanodine receptor 2, an important regulator of calcium (Ca) release from the sarcoplasmic reticulum.[2]

Once the clinical diagnosis of CPVT is made, therapy should be initiated immediately, even without genetic confirmation because the risk for sudden death is high. Nonselective beta blockers such as nadolol are first-line therapy.[3–6] Flecainide, a RYR2 inhibitor, is added to help suppress arrhythmias[1,4,7] and can be especially effective at suppressing VTs during EST. Left cardiac sympathetic denervation can be considered in patients with suboptimal response to medical therapy.[1,4,7,8] Implantable cardioverter defibrillator (ICD) implantation is an option, particularly for noncompliant patients at risk for life-threatening events; however, it is important to approach programming cautiously, by using extended detection times because the potential risks for device and shock-related complications are not insignificant. Inappropriate and even appropriate discharges result in adrenergic stimulation, triggering VT storm; death has occurred despite having a functioning ICD in place.[1,3,4,7] Serial EST and continual monitoring with implantable loop recorders can be used to assure adequate therapy and monitor patient compliance.[9] This patient was ultimately treated with nadolol, flecainide, and an implantable loop recorder (ILR) without an ICD. He has been fully compliant with antiarrhythmic medications and has remained asymptomatic.

CASE 2: CLINICAL PRESENTATION

A 17-year-old asymptomatic boy presented for sports clearance. His ECG revealed nonspecific ST-T wave abnormalities and prolonged corrected QT interval (QTc) of 619 milliseconds with prominent U waves (**Fig. 2**A), prompting cardiac evaluation. His echocardiogram was normal. PVC and slow polymorphic VT were seen at baseline and while actively exercising on his EST (see **Fig. 2**B). His ambulatory Holter monitor revealed frequent polymorphic PVCs and bidirectional VT throughout the day, including sleep hours, and accounted for 6% of total beats (see **Fig. 2**C, D). There were notable findings on physical examination (**Fig. 3**). His family history was significant for his mother dying at age 31 years. She presented for a routine health examination at age 30 and was found to have an irregular rhythm. She was sent to an emergency room where she was found to have recalcitrant VT. She never had cardiac symptoms or syncope. Due to recurrent VT, she ultimately underwent a heart transplant, and died from complications 1 year later. A family photo is shown (see **Fig. 3**).

CASE 2: CLINICAL QUESTIONS

1. What is different about this patient's presentation compared to Case 1? Is he at higher risk for arrhythmogenic sudden death?
2. Which significant physical features guide you toward the diagnosis?
3. Would you be surprised if this patient complained of muscle weakness and episodes of falling?
4. Should his arrhythmias be treated if he is asymptomatic?

CASE 2: DISCUSSION

The patient's physical examination is notable for short stature (less than first centile), slightly low set ears, a broad forehead, dental crowding, and very mild fifth finger clinodactyly (see **Fig. 3**A, B). Although mild, the presence of these features confirms the clinical diagnosis. Evaluating the mouth for dental crowding can be helpful and asking about a history of muscle weakness or episodes or falling down or inability to walk (periodic paralysis) can help. Importantly, although periodic paralysis is a distinguishing feature of this disease, not all patients (including this patient) have paralysis symptoms. Genetic testing revealed a heterozygous pathogenic variant in the *KCNJ2* gene.

This is a rare disease called Andersen-Tawil syndrome (ATS) that should be recognized by its unique clinical features. ATS is caused by loss-of-function variants in KCNJ2, which encodes Kir2.1, the inward rectifying potassium channel responsible for regulating the resting membrane potentials in cardiac cells, skeletal muscle fibers, and ectodermal tissue. ATS is an autosomal dominant (AD) disorder characterized by a triad of (1) VAs, (2) periodic paralysis, and (3) distinctive craniofacial and skeletal dysmorphic features. Although the characteristic triad is seen in 60% to 80% of patients with ATS, there is a high degree of phenotypic variability, even among members of the same family. Rarely, however, does any one feature occur in isolation, so it is incumbent on the physician to conduct a thorough history and physical.

As illustrated by the case, the cardiac phenotype includes QT prolongation with prominent U waves on surface ECG, ventricular ectopy, and/or VT on ambulatory monitoring. Because of their propensity for VA, patients with ATS are at risk

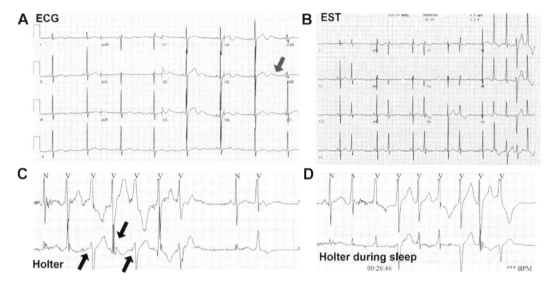

Fig. 2. Documented arrhythmias Case 2. (*A*) The baseline ECG has prominent U waves contributing to a markedly prolonged QTc of 619 ms (*red arrow*). (*B*) During the EST, although at rest, there is slow polymorphic VT. (*C* and *D*) The Holter monitor reveals nonsustained bidirectional VT (*black arrows*) and polymorphic VT during hours consistent with sleep.

for life-threatening arrhythmic events (1.1%/year) and may not have as benign a prognosis as previously believed[10]; those with a history of sustained VT have an increased risk of life-threatening arrhythmic events. Nevertheless, the risk of sudden death in ATS is significantly less than that in CPVT. Notably, VA in ATS frequently occurs at rest, irrespective of adrenergic activation. This

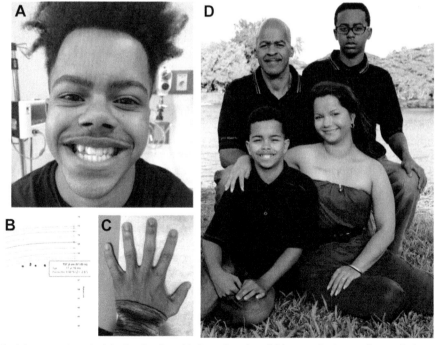

Fig. 3. Clinical features Case 2. (*A*) The forehead is broad with mild hypertelorism and crowded teeth. (*B*) The patient is short statured (less than first centile) and (*C*) has very mild fifth finger clinodactyly. (*D*) The family photo shows the patient in the bottom row next to his mother. His clinical features are mild. His mother may also have mild features consistent with the same diagnosis.

may explain why beta-adrenergic blocking agents lack efficacy in suppressing the arrhythmias. Ventricular ectopy is not always seen during initial clinical evaluation, and hence, patients warrant continued follow-up in cardiology. Sodium channel blockers such as flecainide and propafenone have proven more effective in reducing the arrhythmia burden.[11] This patient has successfully been managed using flecainide.

The extracardiac manifestations of ATS are equally important to its diagnosis and may prompt the first medical referral. In addition to dental abnormalities, craniofacial features may include broad forehead, broad nasal bridge, hypertelorism, low set ears, and micrognathia. Musculoskeletal dysmorphisms such as clinodactyly of the fifth finger, syndactyly of the second and third toes, short stature, and scoliosis may also exist. Periodic paralysis, the final component of the ATS triad, present as episodes of muscle weakness and paralysis occurring spontaneously following prolonged rest or rest after exertion. Episodes can last from hours to days. Carbonic anhydrous inhibitors, such as acetazolamide, can be used for treatment. Muscle strength may or may not fully recover between episodes but muscle weakness becomes permanent over time.[12]

CASE 3: CLINICAL PRESENTATION

An 11-year-old boy collapsed to the ground while casually walking with friends, suffering a cardiac arrest. Full details regarding this case have been previously published.[13] He required CPR and defibrillation and was admitted following successful resuscitation. While in the hospital, his baseline rhythm was noted to be sinus bradycardia with a prolonged QTc of 480 milliseconds. He developed several episodes of polymorphic VT stimulated by adrenergic states, particularly during periods of

irritability and while receiving dobutamine (**Fig.** 4A). Echocardiogram and cardiac MRI demonstrated a structurally normal heart with normal biventricular systolic function and no evidence of fibrosis. His family history was benign with the exception that he was the product of consanguinity. He made a full recovery; he was treated with nadolol and underwent dualchamber transvenous ICD implantation before discharge. Three weeks after discharge, he underwent an EST resulting in the rhythm shown (see **Fig.** 4B). His nadolol dose was doubled and flecainide was added until no further complex ectopy was provoked on EST. Cardiac evaluation of his older brother revealed inducible nonsustained bidirectional VT, without QTc prolongation. Despite an excellent response to nadolol therapy, flecainide was also added empirically for his brother. Unfortunately, despite medication compliance, his brother later died suddenly while playing soccer. Gene sequencing using a commercially available arrhythmia panel yielded negative results; however, based on his history, clinical testing, and family history, a diagnosis was suspected (see "Case 3: discussion" section).

CASE 3: CLINICAL QUESTIONS

1. All 3 cases have documented bidirectional VT. How does this case differ from cases 1 and 2?
2. What is your differential diagnosis and what disease do you think was suspected when genetic testing yielded negative results?

CASE 3: DISCUSSION

Because of the proband's overlapping clinical phenotype of long QT syndrome (LQTS) and CPVT, family history of consanguinity, similarly affected brother, and asymptomatic parents, an

A

B

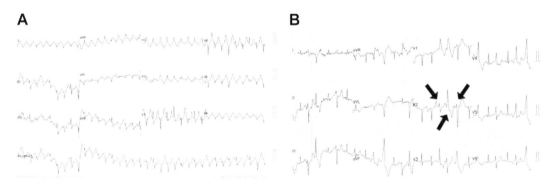

Fig. 4. Case 3: ECG documenting VT while on dobutamine (*A*) and bidirectional VT while running during EST (*B*, *black arrows*). Ebrahim, MA, Alkhabbaz, AA, Albash, B, AlSayegh, AH, Webster, G. Trans-2,3-enoyl-CoA reductase-like-related catecholaminergic polymorphic ventricular tachycardia with regular ventricular tachycardia and response to flecainide. J Cardiovasc Electrophysiol. 2023; 34: 1996-2001. doi:10.1111/jce.16011.

autosomal recessive (AR) disorder causing a less common form of adrenergically stimulated VT was suspected. Although an AR disorder was suspected, the differential diagnosis included syndromes caused by pathogenic variants inherited in both an AD and AR manner including the following: *CALM1-3* (AD/AR), *RYR2* (AD, loss of function), *CASQ2* (AD/AR), TRDN (AR), and trans-2,3-enoyl-CoA reductase-like (TECRL; AR). The initial genetic sequencing for this patient included all genes with the exception of *TECRL*, and thus the *TECRL* gene was suspected. Through whole exome sequencing, known homozygous pathogenic variants in *TECRL* were confirmed in the patient and his brother.[14,15]

To date, only 17 families have been described with *TECRL* variants. Specifically, most reported *TECRL* homozygous variants present during adrenergic stimuli.[13,15,16] *TECRL* plays a key role in intracellular Ca balance.[16] Cell lines affected by *TECRL* abnormalities show downregulation of RYR2 and CASQ2.[16] Treatment of *TECRL*-related arrhythmias remain unclear although most literature supports the use of nonselective beta blockers and flecainide, both used in this patient.[15] This patient exhibited both prolonged QTc and bidirectional VT but standard arrhythmia panels designed to identify genes associated with these traits would yield negative results. This case highlights the necessity of recognizing the clinical symptoms and phenotypes of rare genetic disorders that carry a high mortality risk from life-threatening events.

DISCUSSION AND SUMMARY OF 3 CASES: EVALUATING BIDIRECTIONAL VENTRICULAR TACHYCARDIA

Bidirectional VT is a very specific arrhythmia and should be recognized. The differential diagnosis is limited and includes typical and atypical forms of CPVT, ATS, and digoxin toxicity. Although digoxin toxicity is often obvious through history taking, ATS and CPVT may be more challenging to diagnose.

The main features distinguishing ATS from CPVT are the associated dysmorphic features, periodic paralysis, and the frequent resting VTs in ATS (**Fig. 5**). Yet, as was seen in Case 2, the features of ATS can be mild. One of the most helpful features in differentiating genetic diseases with bidirectional VT is detailed observation of the arrhythmias and the frequency with which they occur. In all 3 cases, patients tend to have sinus bradycardia. However, in classic RYR2 gain of function CPVT, the QTc is generally normal. The QTc may be prolonged in ATS and *TECRL*-related disease but, in ATS, the T wave often has a prominent U wave, which is a valuable clue. Another distinguishing feature is that only classic CPVT

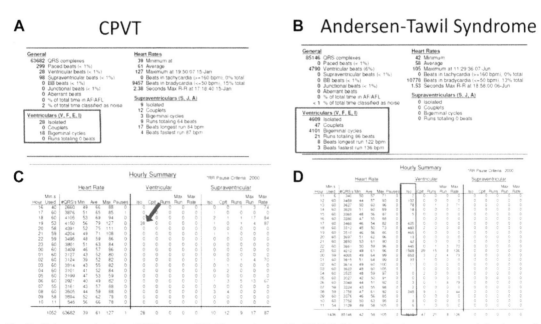

Fig. 5. Holter monitoring, CPVT versus ATS. The patient with CPVT (left) typically demonstrates minimal ventricular ectopy as shown (*A*). There were 28 PVCs all of which occurred in the hour with maximal heart rates (*C, red arrow*). In contrast, the patient with ATS demonstrates high ventricular ectopy burden (6% total) occurring throughout the day, even during sleep (*B, D*).

tends to have AT (see **Fig. 1**). Hence the presence of bidirectional VT and AT during adrenergic stimulation is pathognomonic for CPVT. Finally, Holter monitoring can provide valuable insights (see **Fig. 5**). Patients with CPVT with gain of function variants in *RYR2* tend to have no or minimal ectopy at rest; ectopy or VT only occurs during elevated heart rates. In contrast, in ATS, ectopy and VT tends to occur at rest and even during sleep. These differences in Holter monitor findings between CPVT and ATS are shown in **Fig. 5**. Notice that the rare ectopy seen in the CPVT patient occurs exclusively in a bigeminal pattern, and only during a 1-hour period when the heart rate is the highest. This contrasts with the patient with ATS who has ectopy and VT throughout the 24-hour recording. Family history and genetic testing will also aid clinicians in reaching the diagnosis. That notwithstanding, correctly diagnosing these rare disorders can be challenging if the clinician is not familiar with the differential diagnosis, clinical history, and associated arrhythmias.

CLINICS CARE POINTS

- CPVT is often a missed diagnosis and relies heavily on physicians listening carefully to the clinical history and asking detailed questions surrounding any syncopal event even if seemingly at rest.

- Anxiety, excitement and fear can occur at rest and questions should be directed to elicit if these were present at the time of any syncopal event.

- In a patient with suspected diagnosis of CPVT, clinical testing must include an exercise stress test.

- TECRL gene testing is not available on all commercial panels at the current time. Until it is added, physicians must be alert to add this to testing if TECRL-related disease is suspected.

DISCLOSURE

Mohammad Ebrahim: none; Tam Dan Pham: none; Mary Niu: none; Christina Miyake: none.

ACKNOWLEDGMENT

Christina Miyake is funded by NHLBI K23HL136932. Martin Tristani-Firouzi has several funding sources.

REFERENCES

1. Priori SG, Wilde AA, Horie M, et al. HRS/EHRA/APHRS expert consensus statement on the diagnosis and management of patients with inherited primary arrhythmia syndromes: document endorsed by HRS, EHRA, and APHRS in May 2013 and by ACCF, AHA, PACES, and AEPC in June 2013. Heart Rhythm 2013;10(12):1932–63.

2. Priori SG, Chen SW. Inherited dysfunction of sarcoplasmic reticulum Ca2+ handling and arrhythmogenesis. Circ Res 2011;108(7):871–83.

3. Ackerman MJ, Priori SG, Willems S, et al. HRS/EHRA expert consensus statement on the state of genetic testing for the channelopathies and cardiomyopathies: this document was developed as a partnership between the Heart Rhythm Society (HRS) and the European Heart Rhythm Association (EHRA). Europace 2011;13(8):1077–109.

4. Councils E. 2015 ESC Guidelines for the management of patients with ventricular arrhythmias and the prevention of sudden cardiac death. Eur Heart J 2015;36:2793–867.

5. Leren IS, Saberniak J, Majid E, et al. Nadolol decreases the incidence and severity of ventricular arrhythmias during exercise stress testing compared with β1-selective β-blockers in patients with catecholaminergic polymorphic ventricular tachycardia. Heart Rhythm 2016;13(2):433–40.

6. Peltenburg PJ, Kallas D, Bos JM, et al. An international multicenter cohort study on β-blockers for the treatment of symptomatic children with catecholaminergic polymorphic ventricular tachycardia. Circulation 2022;145(5):333–44.

7. Priori SG, Mazzanti A, Santiago DJ, et al. Precision medicine in catecholaminergic polymorphic ventricular tachycardia: JACC focus seminar 5/5. J Am Coll Cardiol 2021;77(20):2592–612.

8. De Ferrari GM, Dusi V, Spazzolini C, et al. Clinical management of catecholaminergic polymorphic ventricular tachycardia: the role of left cardiac sympathetic denervation. Circulation 2015;131(25):2185–93.

9. Avari Silva JN, Bromberg BI, Emge FK, et al. Implantable loop recorder monitoring for refining management of children with inherited arrhythmia syndromes. J Am Heart Assoc 2016;5(6):e003632.

10. Mazzanti A, Guz D, Trancuccio A, et al. Natural history and risk stratification in andersen-tawil syndrome type 1. J Am Coll Cardiol 2020;75(15):1772–84. https://doi.org/10.1016/j.jacc.2020.02.033.

11. Caballero R, Dolz-Gaiton P, Gomez R, et al. Flecainide increases Kir2.1 currents by interacting with cysteine 311, decreasing the polyamine-induced rectification. Proc Natl Acad Sci U S A 2010;107(35):15631–6. https://doi.org/10.1073/pnas.1004021107.

12. Statland JM, Fontaine B, Hanna MG, et al. Review of the diagnosis and treatment of periodic paralysis. Muscle Nerve 2018;57(4):522–30. https://doi.org/10.1002/mus.26009.

13. Ebrahim MA, Alkhabbaz AA, Albash B, et al. Trans-2, 3-enoyl-CoA reductase-like-related catecholaminergic polymorphic ventricular tachycardia with regular ventricular tachycardia and response to flecainide. J Cardiovasc Electrophysiol 2023. https://doi.org/10.1111/jce.16011.

14. Devalla HD, Gélinas R, Aburawi EH, et al. TECRL, a new life-threatening inherited arrhythmia gene associated with overlapping clinical features of both LQTS and CPVT. EMBO Mol Med 2016;8(12): 1390–408.

15. Webster G, Aburawi EH, Chaix MA, et al. Life-threatening arrhythmias with autosomal recessive TECRL variants. EP Europace 2021;23(5):781–8.

16. Charafeddine F, Assaf N, Ismail A, et al. Novel trans-2, 3-enoyl-CoA reductase–like variant associated with catecholaminergic polymorphic ventricular tachycardia type 3. HeartRhythm Case Reports 2023;9(3):171–7.

Pediatric and Familial Genetic Arrhythmia Syndromes: SCN5A-Related Disorders When It Is Not Long QT Type 3: Clinical Signs and Symptoms

Stephanie F. Chandler, MD[a], Gregory Webster, MD, MPH[a], Christina Y. Miyake, MD, MS[b],*

KEYWORDS

• SCN5A • Brugada syndrome • Overlap • Cardiomyopathy • Conduction block • Atrial standstill

KEY POINTS

- *SCN5A*-related disease causes a diverse set of cardiac conditions including sinus node dysfunction, atrial fibrillation, atrial standstill (AS), long QT syndrome, dilated cardiomyopathy, and Brugada syndrome (BrS).
- Infants and those with biallelic disease can have more severe disease.
- In younger children, ECGs can demonstrate important clinical features that can make the diagnosis even if the child is as of yet asymptomatic. Bradycardia, PR prolongation, and conduction delays are common.
- AS is a feature of SCN5A-related disease and has important implications. Device placement can be challenging and if no atrial depolarization can be achieved, patients are at risk for thromboembolic strokes.

INTRODUCTION

Pediatric and adult patients with SCN5A disease-causing variants often present as overlap syndromes, predominantly with loss-of-function phenotypes. These phenotypes include sick sinus syndrome (SSS), cardiac conduction disease (CCD), isolated Brugada syndrome (BrS), and ventricular arrhythmias (VAs), but more rare phenotypes including atrial standstill (AS) can occur. This series of three case presentations serves to highlight some of the pediatric manifestations of SCN5A disease-causing variants and help clinicians identify patterns of inheritance, better understand clinical features of these diseases, and review potential management strategies.

CASE 1: CLINICAL PRESENTATION

An 8-year-old asymptomatic boy was incidentally found to have a pathogenic truncating SCN5A variant as part of a neurology workup for autism spectrum disorder. His echocardiogram was normal. His ECG had a prolonged PR interval (186 millisecond) and nonspecific intraventricular conduction delay (QRS duration [QRSd] 112 millisecond) (**Fig. 1**A). Four months later, he presented to the emergency room with a fever and his ECG

[a] Division of Cardiology, Ann & Robert H. Lurie Children's Hospital of Chicago, Northwestern University Feinberg School of Medicine, 225 East Chicago Avenue, Box 21, Chicago, IL 60611, USA; [b] Department of Pediatrics, Division of Cardiology, Texas Children's Hospital and Baylor College of Medicine, 6651 Main Street, Houston, TX 77003, USA
* Corresponding author
E-mail address: cymiyake@bcm.edu

Card Electrophysiol Clin 16 (2024) 211–218
https://doi.org/10.1016/j.ccep.2023.10.007

A   **B**

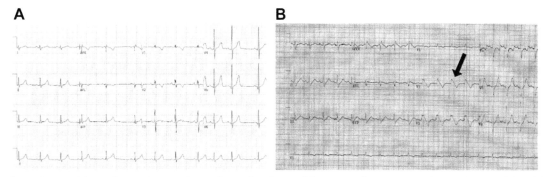

Fig. 1. Case 1. (*A*) Baseline ECG. Note the prolonged PR interval for age and intraventricular conduction delay. (*B*) ECG during fever. Note the type 1 Brugada pattern in anterior precordial leads V2 and V3 (not seen at baseline).

revealed a type 1 Brugada pattern (see **Fig. 1**B). He was admitted until his illness resolved and his ECG had returned to baseline. Several months later, he was evaluated for staring spells. Neurology diagnosed a seizure disorder, but EEG recordings did not fully support the clinical symptoms. An implantable loop monitor (ILR) was placed. Two years later, he had a witnessed syncopal event. His ILR revealed an 8-second sinus pause for which a dual-chamber pacemaker was placed. Since device placement he has remained asymptomatic.

Case 1: Clinical Questions and Important Take-Away Points from This Case

1. *What should I look for in the ECG?* Evaluating ECGs closely is important in identifying SCN5A-related disease in childhood. In the absence of a type 1 Brugada pattern, early evidence of disease includes sinus bradycardia, PR prolongation, and conduction delays (prolonged QRS duration for age).
2. *What are triggers for BrS in children?* Fever is the most common trigger of arrhythmias in young children and can elicit a type 1 Brugada pattern on ECG in some, but not all, children. As a standard approach, children with pathogenic or suspected putative SCN5A variants should be evaluated during a first febrile illness. VAs can be triggered by fevers, so inpatient monitoring should be considered in the setting of a Brugada pattern during febrile illness or if the fever cannot be controlled at home despite antipyretics. Adults, and particularly males, are more likely to have symptoms and cardiac events from BrS.[1,2] In most children, no treatment other than aggressive fever control and avoiding Brugada triggers is required. In children, management focuses on aggressive fever control, avoiding Brugada triggers, and close monitoring for development

of arrhythmias and symptoms. Specifically, it is important to avoid diphenhydramine (Benadryl) and fexofenadine (Allegra), common over-the-counter medications. If children remain febrile despite aggressive use of antipyretics, admission until defervescence is achieved should be considered.
3. *What are typical symptoms?* It is important to be vigilant about symptoms that could be consistent with arrhythmias, particularly in children that demonstrate type 1 Brugada pattern.

CASE 2: CLINICAL PRESENTATION

A 2-month-old girl was delivered urgently at 32 weeks due to in-utero closure of the PDA. Postnatally, her echocardiogram showed severely depressed biventricular function. Her initial ECG demonstrated sinus bradycardia (100 bpm), first-degree AV block (PR 164 millisecond), right atrial enlargement, and a left bundle branch block pattern (**Fig. 2**A). During her hospital course, she developed several episodes of wide complex tachycardia (see **Fig. 2**C, D) and QRS morphology changes due to (1) atrial tachycardia and (2) ventricular tachycardia (VT) (see **Fig. 2**D) and sinus rhythm with rate-related aberrancy (see **Fig. 2**B). Rapid trio whole-exome sequencing revealed a paternally inherited heterozygous pathogenic SCN5A variant previously associated with BrS.

To treat her tachyarrhythmias, atenolol was first chosen due to concerns of sodium channel blocking properties of propranolol. In succession, atenolol, quinidine, sotalol, and propranolol were trialed and discontinued due to worsening conduction delay and persistent salvos of VT. Ultimately, atenolol monotherapy was restarted but due to incomplete VT control, she underwent epicardial dual-chamber implantable cardiac defibrillator (ICD).

The patient family history, including her father who harbored the same SCN5A variant, was

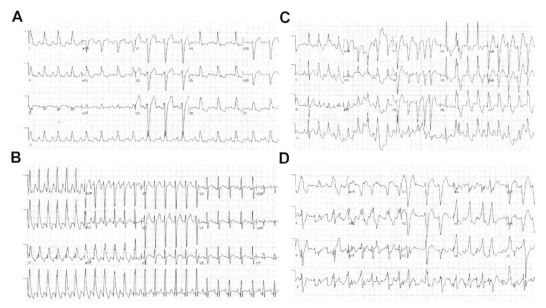

Fig. 2. Case 2. Varying ECGs are shown. Baseline ECG demonstrates sinus bradycardia with prolonged PR interval, right atrial enlargement, and left bundle branch block (*A*). Rate-related aberrant conduction was noted intermittently with varying degrees of intraventricular delay (*A–D*) as well as ventricular tachycardia (*D*).

benign. The youngest of three children, her two older brothers (ages 3 and 7 years) were brought in for cascade screening including clinical evaluation and genetic testing. The diagnosis was suspected in only one of her brothers based on the ECG alone, later confirmed by genetic testing. The brothers' ECGs are shown (**Fig. 3**).

Case 2: Clinical Questions and Important Take-Away Points from This Case

1. *Why should cascade screening be performed?* Pathogenic variants in SCN5A genes are inherited in an autosomal dominant manner and exhibit variable penetrance and expressivity even within the same family. Cascade screening is important to identify other at-risk individuals. Owing to early and severe presentation of the infant, both brothers underwent clinical evaluation in addition to genetic testing. The ECG helped identify one of the brothers as a likely carrier of the familial SCN5A variant (PR prolongation and a mild conduction delay, see **Fig. 3**A), providing an opportunity for counseling even before diagnosis was ultimately confirmed through genetic testing.

2. *What are the signs of SCN5A in an infant?* Infants with SCN5A can present with severe arrhythmias. The combination of sinus node dysfunction (SND), first-degree AV block, conduction block, atrial and VAs, and cardiomyopathy should raise suspicion for SCN5A-related disease. Any degree of ventricular dysfunction in patients with pathogenic SCN5A variants should be followed serially over time.

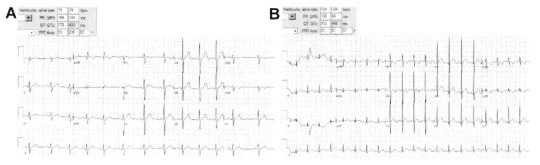

Fig. 3. Case 2. ECGs from two asymptomatic brothers are shown. The ECG in (*A*) a 7-year-old boy and (*B*) a 3-year-old boy. Diagnosis was suspected in one brother based on his ECG, later confirmed when genetic testing returned.

3. *How are arrhythmias treated in children?* In infants, beta blockers may be useful in managing VAs, particularly when rate-related aberrancy is present. Propranolol has partial sodium channel blocking effects and should be used cautiously, as its use may worsen arrhythmias due to the underlying loss of function of the sodium channel. Quinidine is also a standard treatment option for SCN5A-related arrhythmias, although was not effective in this infant. The use of ICDs is complex and can be fraught with complications in the young, including inappropriate shocks, lead fractures, and repeated operations; however, in the absence of dependable pharmacotherapy, device therapy should be considered.

CASE 3: CLINICAL PRESENTATION

A 10-year-old asymptomatic boy presented with bradycardia. His initial ECG demonstrated junctional rhythm (56 bpm) (**Fig. 4**A) with no evidence of atrial depolarization and a normal QTc. His echocardiogram demonstrated a structurally normal heart with normal biventricular size and function. A Holter monitor demonstrated 444 pauses (longest 5.5 seconds, **Fig. 5**A), nonsustained usual complex tachycardia suspected to be junctional (see **Fig. 5**B), and frequent premature ventricular contractions accounting for 2% of total beats.

Family history revealed his father had died in a single-car accident. His father's medical history included a prior cardioversion during a febrile illness. His paternal grandfather had died in his sleep at age 52 from an unknown etiology. Genetic testing revealed two heterozygous missense variants in SCN5A: one classified as pathogenic and the other likely pathogenic.

Owing to marked pauses, the patient was taken to the electrophysiology laboratory for device placement. An electroanatomical map was created to assess atrial and ventricular voltages to prepare for device placement because both sensing and capture can be challenging in these cases.[3] The electrophysiology (EP) study

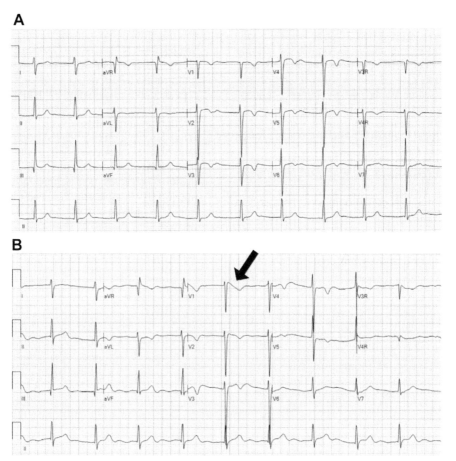

Fig. 4. Case 3. (*A*) Baseline ECG shows a junctional rhythm with intraventricular conduction delay. No *P* waves are seen. (*B*) ECG during fever demonstrate ST elevation in V1 consistent with type 1 Brugada pattern.

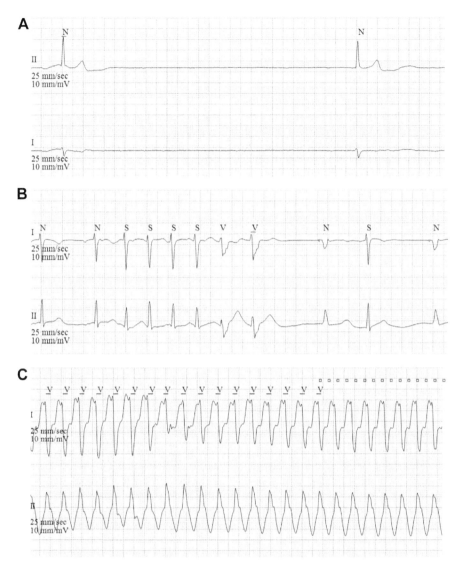

Fig. 5. Case 3. Arrhythmias typical in SCN5A are noted. (*A*) There is a prolonged almost 6 second pause. No atrial activity is seen, consistent with atrial standstill. (*B*) Non-sustained runs of usual complex, suspected junctional tachycardia. (*C*) Ventricular tachycardia.

demonstrated AS (no atrial activity in the right heart) and patchy areas of low voltages with elevated capture threshold in the right. Programmed ventricular stimulation reproducibly induced non-sustained monomorphic VT. A single-chamber ICD was implanted because atrial capture could not be achieved. During the procedure, the patient's body temperature increased to 39.2°C which induced monomorphic VT (see **Fig. 5**C). Neither isoproterenol nor esmolol terminated the VT and active cooling with ice was used to bring down the body temperature. Ultimately, the VT was terminated with rapid ventricular pacing using the newly placed right ventricle

(RV) lead. An ECG while febrile revealed a subtle type I Brugada pattern (see **Fig. 4**B). Owing to AS, anticoagulation was started for stroke prevention and metoprolol and quinidine were used to treat the atrial and VAs.

Owing to concerning family history of suspected BrS, the family underwent cascade screening. Positive results for the pathogenic variant in the paternal aunt and negative results in the paternal grandmother confirmed the patient's father and paternal grandfather harbored the same variant. The patient's mother harbored the second likely pathogenic variant, confirming the patient had compound heterozygous variants in trans, likely contributing to his more severe disease including AS.

Case 3: Clinical Questions and Important Take-Away Points from This Case

1. *How did genetic testing prove the patient's father and grandfather harbored the same pathogenic variant?* Genetic testing and cascade screening are critical to identify at-risk individuals and can be useful to help determine obligate carriers among family members even if deceased. An obligate carrier is determined to harbor a familial variant based on family testing. As an example, in this case, the patient's father is an obligate carrier because the only way his son (the patient) and the patient's aunt (the father's sister) harbor the same gene is if the father passes the variant to his child. Because two siblings (the father and his sister) harbored the same variant, one of their parents had to have passed it to them. Because the grandmother is negative, then the grandfather (who suspiciously died in his sleep) had to have harbored the variant.

2. *What is meant by variants in "trans"*: Because each person has two copies of each chromosome, the term cis or trans is used if two different variants in the same gene are located on the same (cis) or different (trans) alleles. This is an important point in managing patients because two different (ie, compound heterozygous) variants are more likely to cause disease if in trans, because neither chromosome will produce a normal protein. If you can prove two pathogenic variants are inherited from each parent, you can confirm they are in trans which has implications for more severe disease. In this case, genetic testing was able to determine that he inherited one variant from each parent. The use of genetic testing in such manner can help in making a diagnosis.

3. *Why is it important to diagnose AS?* Patients with AS and without the capacity for atrial pacing are at risk for thromboembolic events and warrant anticoagulation.[4,5] In addition to lack of atrial depolarization, ventricular sensing and thresholds can be compromised. This raises two important clinical considerations. First, during device implant, even ventricular lead placement can be challenging due to elevated ventricular thresholds. Second, even after successful implant, ventricular thresholds can fluctuate particularly during fever, resulting in loss of capture and syncope if the patient is pacemaker-dependent. Compound heterozygous variants in the SCN5A gene may be more likely to present with AS.[3,4]

SUMMARY DISCUSSION OF THREE PATIENT CASES AND *SCN5A*

The *SCN5A* gene encodes the pore-forming ion conducting alpha subunit of the main cardiac sodium channel NaV1.5. Pathogenic variants in *SCN5A* have been associated with a diverse set of cardiac conditions including SND, atrial fibrillation, AS, long QT syndrome, dilated cardiomyopathy, and BrS. Both loss-and gain-of-function variants are described, whereas occasionally a variant results in functional channels with aspects of both, leading to a disease with overlapping phenotypes.[6] The absence of a genotype–phenotype correlation in families affected by BrS underscores the complexity of this arrhythmogenic entity.[2] Pathogenic SCN5A variants usually show an autosomal dominant inheritance pattern, with variable penetrance, but also recessive forms with homozygous or compound heterozygous mutations are described and can be more severe with pediatric patients at higher risk for Brugada ECG pattern, VAs, and cardiac arrest[3,4,7]

BRUGADA SYNDROME

BrS is a familial arrhythmia classically characterized by ST-elevations in the right precordial leads on ECG. Known external factors promoting arrhythmic events in patients with BrS include fever and specific drugs (www.Brugadadrugs.org).[8] Although usually diagnosed in adults, BrS has been identified in children and infants.[9] Nevertheless, SCN5A variants account for less than 30% of clinically diagnosed BrS patients.

The management of patients with BrS—as with most diagnoses—depends partially on clinical features of the disease. Patients with documented life-threatening VA should be considered as candidates for ICD therapy.[1] Other important findings for risk stratification include a spontaneous type 1 ECG. Management strategies include: aggressive treatment of fever with antipyretic drugs in patients with a clear type 1 ECG and heart rhythm monitoring; avoidance of specific drugs including common over-the counter medications such as diphenhydramine (Benadryl) and fexofenadine (Allegra); and avoidance of excessive alcohol use.[10] Pharmacologic therapy includes quinidine[11] while acute management of arrhythmic storm includes isoproterenol,[1] and in this patient, rapid ventricular pacing was effective. The utility of beta blockers in some patients and infants has been reported in limited small pediatric studies.[12] Finally, and more recently, ablation of the arrhythmogenic substrate in the right ventricular outflow tract—often from an epicardial approach—has demonstrated promising results in some centers with expertise in this form of ablation.[13]

SICK SINUS SYNDROME

SCN5A variants can also present phenotypically as SSS—a disease characterized by sinoatrial node dysfunction. Clinically, this can present as sinus bradycardia, sinus arrest, and reduced chronotropic response.[14] This pathophysiology usually manifests during adulthood—often in association with fibrosis or ischemia; however, there are patients in whom SSS manifests at a much younger age and this has been linked to SCN5A variants.[15,16]

ATRIAL STANDSTILL

AS is a rare condition that is defined as the absence of electrical activity within the cardiac atria. One of the most important observations in pediatric patients with AS is a relatively high rate of major thromboembolic events.[4,5] Also notable, device placement in either atrium or ventricle can be challenging due to poor sensing and elevated capture thresholds that can fluctuate over time, with thresholds potentially increasing during times of fever, resulting in loss of capture.[3,4] In some cases, atrial capture cannot be achieved. If atrial depolarization cannot be achieved, anticoagulation should be considered for stroke prevention.[4,5]

OVERLAP SYNDROMES

Appropriately named due to the presence of different elements of the phenotype found in various combinations in families,[17] the first evidence that a single SCN5A variant can result in multiple phenotypic pathophysiologies came from the description of the 1795insD mutation which was characterized in a large multigenerational Dutch family.[18] In pediatric-specific studies, patients with SCN5A disease causing variants presented mainly as overlap syndromes, with predominant loss-of-function phenotypes of SSS, progressive conduction disease, and VAs.[19] Early age of onset is associated with severity in many genetic diseases.[20] In a large prospective multicenter pediatric cohort of SCN5A variant-positive neonates, it was reported that although 67.9% were asymptomatic at diagnosis, independent risk factors for cardiac events included age less than 1 year at diagnosis, compound heterozygous mutations and mutations with both gain and loss of

function.[21] Compound heterozygosity is usually associated with a more severe phenotype.

In conclusion, pediatric patients with SCN5A disease causing variants can present with an array of clinical phenotypes from asymptomatic to arrhythmogenic syndromes—often as an overlap syndrome, but also with predominantly loss-of-function phenotypes including SSS, CCD, and VAs, but most frequently as an autosomal dominant trait, with variable penetrance and variable expressivity.[22]

DISCLOSURES

Stephanie Chandler, Gregory Webster, Christina Miyake: None.

FUNDING

C. Miyake is funded through NHLBI K23HL136932. G. Webster is funded through NIH, United State/ NHLBI, United State R01 HL164773.

REFERENCES

1. Priori SG, Wilde AA, Horie M, et al. HRS/EHRA/ APHRS expert consensus statement on the diagnosis and management of patients with inherited primary arrhythmia syndromes: document endorsed by HRS, EHRA, and APHRS in May 2013 and by ACCF, AHA, PACES, and AEPC in June 2013. Heart Rhythm 2013;10(12):1932–63.

2. Skinner JR, Winbo A, Abrams D, et al. Channelopathies that lead to sudden cardiac death: clinical and genetic aspects. Heart Lung Circ 2019;28(1): 22–30.

3. Chiang DY, Kim JJ, Valdes SO, et al. Loss-of-Function SCN5A mutations associated with sinus node dysfunction, atrial arrhythmias, and poor pacemaker capture. Circ Arrhythm Electrophysiol 2015;8(5): 1105–12.

4. Howard TS, Chiang DY, Ceresnak SR, et al. Atrial standstill in the pediatric population: a multi-institution collaboration. JACC Clin Electrophysiol 2023;9(1):57–69.

5. Ahnfeldt AM, de Knegt VE, Reimers JI, et al. Atrial standstill presenting as cerebral infarction in a 7-year-old girl. SAGE Open Med Case Rep 2019;7:2050313X19827735. https://doi.org/ 10.1177/2050313X19827735.

6. Remme CA, Verkerk AO, Nuyens D, et al. Overlap syndrome of cardiac sodium channel disease in mice carrying the equivalent mutation of human SCN5A-1795insD. Circulation 2006;114(24):2584–94.

7. Bezzina CR, Rook MB, Groenewegen WA, et al. Compound heterozygosity for mutations (W156X and R225W) in SCN5A associated with severe cardiac conduction disturbances and degenerative

changes in the conduction system. Circ Res 2003; 92(2):159–68.

8. Postema PG, Wolpert C, Amin AS, et al. Drugs and Brugada syndrome patients: review of the literature, recommendations, and an up-to-date website (www.brugadadrugs.org). Heart Rhythm 2009;6(9): 1335–41.

9. Kanter RJ, Pfeiffer R, Hu D, et al. Brugada-like syndrome in infancy presenting with rapid ventricular tachycardia and intraventricular conduction delay. Circulation 2012;125(1):14–22.

10. Ohkubo K, Nakai T, Watanabe I. Alcohol-induced ventricular fibrillation in a case of Brugada syndrome. Europace 2013;15(7):1058.

11. Belhassen B. Management of Brugada syndrome 2016: should all high risk patients receive an ICD? Alternatives to implantable cardiac defibrillator therapy for Brugada syndrome. Circ Arrhythm Electrophysiol. 2016;9(11):1058.

12. Chockalingam P, Wilde AA. Loss-of-function sodium channel mutations in infancy: a pattern unfolds. Circulation 2012;125(1):6–8.

13. Nademanee K. Radiofrequency ablation in Brugada syndrome. Heart Rhythm 2021;18(10):1805–6.

14. Abe K, Machida T, Sumitomo N, et al. Sodium channelopathy underlying familial sick sinus syndrome with early onset and predominantly male characteristics. Circ Arrhythm Electrophysiol. 2014;7(3): 511–7.

15. Yokoi H, Makita N, Sasaki K, et al. Double SCN5A mutation underlying asymptomatic Brugada syndrome. Heart Rhythm 2005;2(3):285–92.

16. Veldkamp MW, Wilders R, Baartscheer A, et al. Contribution of sodium channel mutations to bradycardia and sinus node dysfunction in LQT3 families. Circ Res 2003;92(9):976–83.

17. Remme CA, Wilde AA. SCN5A overlap syndromes: no end to disease complexity? Europace 2008; 10(11):1253–5.

18. Bezzina C, Veldkamp MW, van Den Berg MP, et al. A single Na(+) channel mutation causing both long-QT and Brugada syndromes. Circ Res 1999; 85(12):1206–13.

19. Chen C, Tan Z, Zhu W, et al. Brugada syndrome with SCN5A mutations exhibits more pronounced electrophysiological defects and more severe prognosis: a meta-analysis. Clin Genet 2020;97(1):198–208.

20. Blich M, Khoury A, Suleiman M, et al. Specific therapy based on the genotype in a malignant form of long QT3, carrying the V411M mutation. Int Heart J 2019;60(4):979–82.

21. Baruteau AE, Kyndt F, Behr ER, et al. SCN5A mutations in 442 neonates and children: genotype-phenotype correlation and identification of higher-risk subgroups. Eur Heart J 2018;39(31):2879–87.

22. Villarreal-Molina T, García-Ordóñez GP, Reyes-Quintero Á E, et al. Clinical spectrum of SCN5A channelopathy in children with primary electrical disease and structurally normal hearts. Genes 2021;13(1):16.

Moving?

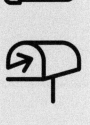

Printed and bound by CPI Group (UK) Ltd, Croydon, CR0 4YY

03/10/2024

01040367-0003